10 Lessons
from a
Former
Fat
Girl

Amy
Parham

HARVEST HOUSE PUBLISHERS

EUGENE, OREGON

Cover by Dugan Design Group, Bloomington, Minnesota

Cover photo © Lolo Highsmith (hair styled by Shannon Peery, Halo Salon, Columbia, SC)

Amy Parham: Published in association with the literary agency of Fedd & Company, Inc., 9759 Concord Pass, Brentwood, TN 37027.

The Biggest Loser is not associated with this book or any of the views or information contained in this book.

10 LESSONS FROM A FORMER FAT GIRL
Copyright © 2010 by Amy Parham
Published by Harvest House Publishers
Eugene, Oregon 97402
www.harvesthousepublishers.com

Library of Congress Cataloging-in-Publication Data
Parham, Amy, 1967-
10 lessons from a former fat girl / Amy Parham.
p. cm.
ISBN 978-0-7369-3865-5 (pbk.)
1. Self-perception—Religious aspects—Christianity. 2. Body image. 3. Health—Religious aspects—Christianity. 4. Women—Religious life. 5. Food—Religious aspects—Christianity. 6. Emotions—Religious aspects—Christianity. I. Title. II. Title: Ten lessons from a former fat girl.
BV4598.25.P37 2011
248.4—dc22

2010025556

Printed in the United States of America

10 11 12 13 14 15 16 17 18 / BP-NI / 10 9 8 7 6 5 4 3 2 1

To all the women who feel like prisoners
in their bodies and long to be free,
this book is dedicated to you.

I would like to thank Jesus Christ, the giver of all freedom. I would also like to thank my husband, Phillip, for being my best friend; my boys, Austin, Pearson, and Rhett, for loving me just the way I am; my daddy, Don Pearson, for loving me with a love that exemplifies the love of Christ; and my mother, Margaret Williams, for showing me how to be a strong woman by being an excellent role model.

Finally, I send big hugs and thanks to all the women who are too numerous to list—but know who they are—for influencing my life in big and small ways and continuing to teach me fit-girl lessons through their examples, words, and deeds.

Contents

Life Is the Journey, Not the Arrival

*All changes, even the most longed for,
have their melancholy; for what we leave
behind us is a part of ourselves; we must die
to one life before we can enter another.*

—ANATOLE FRANCE

Why is everyone so obsessed with their weight? This is the question I started asking myself when I had finally made the decision to settle for being the fat girl. I mean, I had a lot going for me. Why should the extra weight matter? I was organized. I was a great hostess. I volunteered in my church. I was a good wife, mother, and friend. Even though I had ballooned to 240 pounds and was tired all the time, weight was one area I decided to give myself a break. It didn't bother me, so why should it bother anyone else?

I got defensive when family members expressed their concerns and offered helpful suggestions to lose weight. My sister-in-law, who I always thought of as the skinny girl, repeatedly tried to encourage me with my weight loss. I remember one time when she took me out to lunch. As we were getting ready to leave, she presented me with a gift—a food journal. She was very excited about the prospect of teaching me how to write down my food intake each and every day. As you can imagine, I didn't share her enthusiasm. Simply looking at that book exhausted me.

See, I looked at the skinny girl as a different animal from me. I never truly believed that the things that worked for her would work for me. I somehow thought that I was different, and so my body worked differently than hers did. I didn't believe I could ever be like her, so why would I even try? This is the mentality of those of us who have been trapped inside our bodies and minds as fat girls.

Then something happened that changed the course of this fat girl. Along came a television reality show called *The Biggest Loser*. In 2008 my husband and I were chosen out of 300,000 hopeful candidates to go on television and reveal to America our struggle with obesity. This was an amazing opportunity but one that forced me to look at myself in a whole new way. The fat girl was to be exposed, and there was no place to hide from the truth. My husband and I lost a total of 256 pounds together as a couple on that show. That is an amazing victory, but that was just the beginning of the war. The weight-loss process revealed deeper issues that had caused us to put on the weight in the first place. Dealing with these issues would become the real challenge and the thing that solidified the transformation from the fat girl to the fit girl.

That is why this book may be different from any weight-loss book you have ever read. This book talks about not only the physical aspects of weight loss, but also the very real mental and emotional challenges that exist. It's about learning how to transform a fat girl (a woman who has poor eating and exercise habits, a food addiction, a lack of self-esteem, and a distorted image of herself, God, and others) into a fit girl (a woman who practices healthy eating and exercise habits, takes care of herself emotionally, physically, and mentally, and believes in herself and God).

This book is about identifying those areas in your life where you've held yourself back from becoming the woman God created you to be. It's about digging up roots of bitterness and unforgiveness in your heart. It's about releasing those people and things in your past that have hurt you and, by doing so, gaining freedom from compulsions that rule your life. We have all been on a million diets, but have we dealt with the roots of our problems? For me, I had tried every diet I could find, but I never had focused on the core of the problem.

Be assured that this book is not a diet book or a manual to make you as skinny as a supermodel in 45 days or less. It is not a get-fit-quick scheme or program. I am not promoting any pills, potions, or magic fairy dust that you must buy now to change your life by tomorrow. I am not selling you an unrealistic expectation or a promise that the journey toward becoming a fit girl is an easy one. In fact, it's quite the opposite. It's a tough process and requires the peeling back of many layers.

I didn't understand this truth early on in my weight-loss journey. In my case, the more weight I lost (I lost more than 100 pounds), the more I realized that if I was really going to transform myself permanently, then in addition to my physical body, I was going to have to deal with the fat girl that lived on the inside.

What a wake-up call that was! One of the ways I did this was by searching deep inside my soul and figuring out why I was overweight to begin with. It's a shame that while most of us know that diet and exercise are the keys to weight loss, not many of us know the importance about talking about and dealing with the roots of the problem—*why* did we become overweight?

For me, it was an emotional crutch. I had always turned to food in times of stress, sadness, happiness, anger, or just about any emotion. It became instinctual. To further fuel my addiction to food, my parents owned a restaurant and ice-cream parlor. Can you guess what my favorite food was? I'll give you a hint. It's frozen and chocolate. Yep! Ice cream!

You can imagine how spending so much time in the back room of the family restaurant further charged my problem with compulsive eating. These were the realities that I started unraveling as I began to lose weight. It was hard to let go of my emotional-eating crutch. With food no longer acting as my security blanket, I felt like a skydiver who had jumped out of an airplane without a parachute.

I spent much of my life fighting against the fat-girl mentality. She was there even when I was thin. Have you ever looked at a skinny picture of yourself, but all you could see or remember was how fat you were or felt? That's a fat girl living on the inside of the fit girl. Unfortunately, the fat girl wields a lot of power. Time and time again, I would find the willpower to lose some weight and take better care of myself, but after a little success, I would panic and find myself slowly turning and running back to the comforts of my old identity. There was something about the fat girl that I couldn't get rid of. The problem was she was sabotaging my life!

Can you relate? If you have struggled with your relationship with food, your weight, and your body, then you must know that *I am you.* Have you been comforting yourself and celebrating every victory with food? Have you felt like a failure time and time again because you felt like your willpower wasn't strong enough? Me too! It sounds like you need to deal with the fat girl on the inside!

I want to encourage you. You don't have to struggle with your weight forever. You, too, can become a fit girl! Once you deal with the fat girl on the inside and become a fit girl, you will never be the same. You will be able to control impulsive reactions to food. You will see yourself as a different person. You will have more confidence. Isn't that what you want? I know it is because you are reading this book.

Whenever my friends and I embark on a new adventure, challenge, project, or life change, we chant in unison, "Life is the journey and not the arrival!" Saying this reminds us that life happens in the moments and through the process, not necessarily in the outcome. In the same sense, this journey of saying no to the fat girl and yes to the fit girl is a process and not an event. It is good to create goals and work toward them, but don't forget the important lessons are found in the journey.

This journey is one of the most difficult yet rewarding adventures you will ever take. I love this quote from Donald Miller's book *Blue Like Jazz*: "It is always the simple things that change our lives. And these things never happen when you are looking for them to happen. Life will reveal answers at the pace life wishes to do so. You feel like running, but life is on a stroll. This is how God does things." This is reminiscent of the journey to becoming the fit girl. You think it is all about losing weight, and then God slowly, in His own way, reveals something that will change your life from the inside out.

Hopefully, what you will read about in these pages will help you examine your life in a new way and, if necessary, motivate you to make some changes. Change is usually not easy. That is why they are called growing pains. That is why when you work out with weights and build muscle, it hurts. That is why childbirth is painful. Anything worthwhile in life requires work, sacrifice, and usually pain. Are you willing to work through the pain to find the fit girl inside of you? Come with me. I want to help you find her.

> Any change, even a change for the better, is always accompanied by drawbacks and discomforts. —Arnold Bennett

Before we get started, find a notebook or journal so you can record some of the thoughts and feelings you have as you read this book. You can also use the space at the end of each chapter for this purpose. At the end of each chapter, you will also find a "Transformation Tips" section that includes questions to meditate on and answer. Use your notebook or the space provided to jot down the answers and thoughts to the questions.

There's just one more thing to explain. For me, prayer is super important. I close each chapter with a section titled "Your Prayer." Take the time to pray this short prayer. It will help stimulate your faith during this journey and give you strength where you need it most.

Now let's go find your fit-girl self!

Lesson 1

We All Have an Empty Place

*We're all searching for something to fill up what I like
to call that big, God-shaped hole in our souls. Some
people use alcohol, or sex, or their children, or food, or
money, or music, or heroin. A lot of people even use the
concept of God itself. I could go on and on. I used to
know a girl who used shoes. She had over two-hundred
pairs. But it's all the same thing, really. People, for some
stupid reason, think they can escape their sorrows.*

—Tiffanie DeBartolo, *God-Shaped Hole*

My earliest memories were such happy ones. Mom had dinner on
the table when Dad came home from work, and my three sisters and I laughed and talked about our day with our parents. It was the best feeling. Everything about our family felt so right and secure. I remember Mom walking me to kindergarten every day at a church around the corner from my house. In that same church parking lot, my dad taught me how to ride a bike without training wheels. He also taught me to fly a kite, and with his help, I won a blue ribbon in a kite-flying competition at my school.

I had my own bedroom with a yellow gingham canopy bed and a playhouse in the backyard. There was also a dogwood tree that I climbed all the time. My best friend, Teresa, lived across the street, and my grandparents lived nearby. Life was good and felt normal, but when I turned eight years old, my seemingly perfect life changed forever.

A Growing Hole

Dad quit his longtime job at a local radio station in South Carolina to pursue a job at another radio station in West Palm Beach, Florida. We had to sell our house immediately and move to what seemed to me to be a different planet. I will never forget the image of Teresa and me standing by the "For Sale" sign in our front yard. We bawled our eyes out and held each other so tight because we knew we might not ever see each other again.

When we got to Florida, the five of us moved into a tiny apartment. There was nothing wrong with the apartment, but I was uncomfortable because I was used to living in a larger space and having a big yard to play in. My sisters and I barely had enough room to squeeze past each other on the way to the bathroom. My new school was huge compared to the one I attended in South Carolina. But the worst thing was that while everyone knew and loved me at my old school, I was now the new girl at school, and I got ridiculed for it. I felt insecure, unsure of myself, and alone. I wanted to go back to my happy, carefree life.

This was the first time I remember being unhappy and having no control over my circumstances. I was deeply sad, and it felt like I had an empty hole in my soul. Thankfully, we only stayed in Florida for one year, but things would never go back to how they were before. I would never regain the sense of normalcy I had so desperately craved.

When we came back to South Carolina, we moved to a different city, and my parents bought a restaurant and ice-cream parlor. It was hard work building a new business, and the stress took a toll on Mom and Dad. They began to fight all the time about money and other issues. It got so bad that they divorced.

When my parental situation turned upside down, I found myself in a world that lacked security and stability. Suddenly, I was being raised by a single mother, and as the oldest daughter at ten years old, there was a lot of pressure on me to help my mom care for my two sisters. She worked very hard (sometimes up to 18 hours a day), and I know she did her best to keep food on the table and clothes on our backs. She usually had no time to tuck us in at night and tell us bedtime stories because she worked such long hours.

My sisters (who were four and six years old) and I spent a lot of time at home alone. As much as we tried to pick up after ourselves, you can imagine how messy three kids can be. I felt terrible when my mother would come home, tired from working so much, and be cranky because the house was such a disaster. I never felt like I could do enough to make Mom happy or fix our broken home life.

Many mornings she had to get to work at the crack of dawn and woke us up at three in the morning to take us to the restaurant. She made us a makeshift bed on the concrete floor in the back room and let us sleep there while she worked. This was not an ideal environment for kids, but she was doing the best she could.

It wasn't her fault. The problem was me. I felt the hole inside my heart growing bigger and bigger, and I desperately needed something to fill it.

Enter the Banana Split

I remember one particular day when I was playing outside the restaurant and decided to go visit the couple who worked at the dry cleaners next door. The owners were in their late twenties and had no children of their own. They were kind enough to let me hang out with them sometimes, and it made me feel good.

In my mind, I felt "less than" because my life had changed so drastically in only two years. I was nothing like the other kids at school and always felt out of place. This couple welcomed, accepted, and loved me just the way I was. They talked to me like I was one of their peers, and I appreciated the kindness and warmth they showed me.

This day was like any other day that I would drop by for a visit. I had been sitting at the counter and talking to the wife for about 20 minutes when her husband walked in. He abruptly told me that it was time for me to go. He said that their business was no place for children and that I shouldn't hang out there so much.

I was hurt to my core and very embarrassed. I thought they were my friends, but they were abandoning me. I tried my best to maintain my composure and make myself believe that it didn't matter. I reassured myself that I didn't need them and was fine on my own. I remember announcing to them that I was leaving, anyway, to go to make a banana split for myself.

I guess in my own childlike way, I was trying to hold on to my self-respect by pointing out that I could have a banana split anytime I wanted one. Maybe it seems silly, but for me that moment was a turning point because it concerned food. I ended up making myself that banana split and hoping it would fill some of the rejection and the emptiness I had been feeling for so long. It was the first time I used food for comfort, but it would definitely not be the last time.

Bigger and Bigger

As I got older, I gained weight and came under the attack of my grandmother who constantly told me I was chubby. My two sisters were in this weight battle with me. What else would anyone expect from kids who ate fast food and ice cream every day for years? Being overweight compounded our problems in school. Not only were we still the new kids on the block, but we had also become the fat kids.

My youngest sister had an especially hard time with children teasing her. To this day, she talks about the negative memories—one of which was having to shop for clothes in the husky department at Sears—that have haunted her through the years. Not only did she suffer from a kidney problem that made her gain even more weight, she also had an eye condition and had to wear coke-bottle glasses. She felt like such an outcast, and it broke my heart. At this point, I had taken on the role of surrogate mother for my sisters. I felt responsible for them and believed it was my job to protect them. I hated to see them suffer so much.

I don't say all of this to blame my parents. I know they both loved us girls very much and did their best at the time, but the fact was I felt very alone and abandoned. While my mom worked long hours to support us, my father took up a new life. He started dating a woman soon after the divorce. We didn't realize how serious the relationship was until we found out they had gotten married. My sisters and I weren't even invited to the wedding.

Yet again, I felt I was left behind as he started a whole new life without my sisters and me. This feeling was further reinforced when he purchased a two-seater sports car. I remember thinking that there wasn't enough room for my sisters and me. Where were we going to fit in? To me, the car was a symbol of how we weren't a part of Dad's life anymore.

My void grew deeper with each passing day. As I shoved more food into my mouth to soothe the pain that wouldn't go away, my weight crept up.

When I was eleven years old, my friend Beth invited me to attend her church youth group one night. My grandfather was a Pentecostal preacher, and church was a big part of our lives. We visited many churches through the years and spent many weeks during the summers at different vacation Bible schools, which were hosted by local congregations. I had even accepted Christ into my heart at a young age.

Since moving back to South Carolina, however, our family had stopped going to church. I missed it. The thought of visiting one with my friend absolutely thrilled me. When I arrived at the service, I immediately felt as if I belonged. I was in a wonderful place where people loved and cared about each other. It felt like I was home again. Church became my refuge. I especially felt drawn to the youth pastor, Sam. He quickly became a father figure to me, and I felt like I could tell him anything.

This reconnection with church sparked the beginning of a deepening relationship with God. Every Tuesday night, the church bus would drive to my house and take me to church. It was there that I experienced overwhelming love from others, and I discovered that God wanted to fill up the empty hole inside of my heart.

My faith commitment didn't mean that my problems were suddenly solved. I didn't ride off into the sunset of my new, happily-ever-after future. It just meant that for the first time in a long time, I felt like I had a lifeline. I had hope. My heart had a chance to become whole.

By learning about God's love for me, I realized that because we are all human, we all carry with us a certain measure of hurt and pain. This is a part of the sin nature of humankind. But that was not all. I also discovered that God created us with a space that only He can fill. He wanted to be the one to fill my voids and heal my hurts. The pain I was trying to mask with ice cream was a pain that only He could mend.

The Fat Girl Thinks She Is in Control

I want you to know that emptiness is normal. If you feel as if you need to numb the pain or soothe your soul with something outside of yourself, you are not alone. We all endure suffering from time to time. It's a normal process of living in a sinful world.

While emptiness is normal, it is how you fill the emptiness that will determine whether you are a fat girl or a fit girl. These two chicks cope with problems in different ways. The fit girl chooses God. The fat girl chooses unhealthy addictions. The fat girl can use many different ways to try to heal the hurt on the inside. Some abuse food, drugs, or alcohol or become addicted to work, hobbies, or unhealthy relationships. It might be hard to believe, but some folks can even abuse exercise to an addictive level.

Let me tell you something. The hole that is formed inside of us is not shaped like an ice-cream cone, a vodka bottle, a cigarette, or a good-looking guy. The hole is shaped like the Holy Spirit, the Comforter. He is the one who is meant to fill our empty places and heal our hurts.

I like to think about it this way. We have been created like puzzles with a missing piece. That piece is a relationship with God. He wants us to invite Him into our hearts. The closer we walk with God, the less we will search for other things to fill the hole. This is something the fit girl knows and understands.

I will be honest with you. There have been many times in my life, especially as a fat girl, when I have drifted away from my relationship with the Lord. I'm not a psychiatrist, but I believe that because of the instability I felt as a result of my parent's divorce, I made a decision as a little girl that when I became an adult, I would be self-sufficient. I would take care of myself so that bad things would never happen to me again.

As most of us know, life usually doesn't turn out as smooth as we hope it will. Bad things happen to everyone. Here's a reality check. In life, people will disappoint us one way or another. If you have never been hurt or offended by someone, then you just might be an alien from outer space. The fact is none of us can measure up to perfection, and since we can't, then certainly life will never be perfect.

My sense of independence severely impaired me when it came to trusting God with my life. I voiced my commitment to Him, but when things got tough or trials came my way, I wanted to take back my commitment. I wanted to do things my way instead of His way. When I turned away from God, that original hole in my heart would reappear, and I temporarily filled it with something. My choices were usually food, of course, and sometimes alcohol or the attention of the opposite sex. None of those things ever gave me true contentment because nothing outside of God could fulfill me.

A significant time I pulled away from God was when my son Rhett was diagnosed with autism. I was 35 at the time, and Rhett was 3. Autism is a spectrum disorder that presents different social and psychological abnormalities in some children. The main challenges we had with Rhett were that he screamed nonstop and was very sensitive to certain sounds. He also had a high threshold for pain. If he was hurting, he didn't know how to tell us, and so my husband and I were always afraid that he might be sick and we would never know.

We faced other obstacles with our son. Rhett acted as if he had no fear. He was always jumping off the top of the sliding board, and one time he even climbed out of his bedroom window and onto the roof. He exhibited destructive behaviors, colored on the walls, overfilled the bathroom sink or tub with water, and broke things around the house at random. Because he couldn't communicate in a normal manner, he was easily frustrated.

It was a very sad and dark time in our lives. I was utterly exhausted. I couldn't believe that God would allow my child to be this way, especially because I tried to live a good Christian life. For goodness sake, I even served Him in ministry at church! *Why me?* This was the question I constantly asked myself whenever I threw a pity party, which was quite often. *This should not happen to someone like me,* I thought.

I determined that if my son could suffer from autism when God was supposed to be in control, then maybe I should take back the reins of my life and chart my own course. I would figure out how to fix Rhett. I would find a way to make him better by myself. Who needed God? I was pretty sure I could handle things on my own.

As I focused on being in control, guess what happened? That's right. The hole that formed when my family fell apart grew bigger. And that's when the fat girl came out in full force. When it came time for bed, I was so exhausted from trying to do everything on my own that I would fall into a heap on the sofa. I spent many nights with my new comforters—a bowl of ice cream or a bag of chips. Oh, I still had conversations with God, but they were more like yelling matches. I would demand that He fix Rhett in the spirit of "You got me into this mess, God, so You'd better get me out of it."

One day as I was driving down the road and screaming at God yet again, He gently put me in my place. A still, small voice spoke quietly to my heart and said, "Amy, you aren't perfect, and I love you. Why does Rhett have to be perfect for you to love him?" Talk about getting hit right between the eyes! I knew that God was absolutely right. I was definitely not perfect, and instead of loving Rhett for who he was and dealing with the situation at hand, I had been focusing on making him normal (whatever that even means). At that moment I shifted my focus and asked God to forgive me. I asked Him to help me trust Him with Rhett and the other challenges in my life.

I quickly came to the realization that when I controlled my life, I only made more of a mess of it. It was a lesson I would continue to learn even after I lost the weight and transformed into a fit girl. (By the way, you'll quickly find out that the fit girl is always learning!)

A week later, I was at church, and as I listened to the sermon, the pastor stopped in the middle of what he was saying and told the congregation that he felt led to say something specific. He said that there was someone in the service who didn't know how much longer they could hang on, and that they should be encouraged because God was about to perform a miracle in their life.

I was stunned. Only a few days earlier, I mumbled something to myself about not being able to take these problems anymore. Not only was I dealing with my weight—I was 230 pounds at that point—and Rhett's autism diagnosis, but my husband, Phillip, and I had also lost a business right after we had purchased a home that needed thousands of dollars worth of renovations. I was emotionally drained by these problems. It seemed I couldn't get a break.

I felt as if the pastor was talking to me. It was the encouragement I needed to hear. Maybe my life would get better! Within days, the miracles started happening. First, we found out about a therapy called "audio integration" that proved to be a miracle cure for Rhett. It stopped his sensitivity to sound and his constant screaming. We were able to catch and keep his attention for a long period of time, and for the first time, I felt he could actually begin to learn. Second, our financial situation started to turn around as we found new careers in real estate.

When things started changing for the better, Phil and I specifically realized we had been feeding our physical bodies instead of filling our spiritual bodies. In the process, we had become morbidly obese. It was time to begin the journey to lose the weight. For me, it was time to say good-bye to the fat girl and hello to the fit girl.

What about you? What's your story? I have met people all over the country who have stories that make mine seem like a walk in the park. One such lady that I met recently told me that her problems with her weight began right after her husband committed suicide. That in itself is a horrifying traumatic event, and now this woman is left to pick up the pieces of a family torn apart by tragedy. This affected her and her family emotionally, mentally, and financially. Five years later this lady is obese, depressed, and struggling to support her family. My heart goes out to people like this because I see the magnitude of their holes and how they are desperately trying to fill them.

Pascal wrote, "What else does this craving, and this helplessness, proclaim but that there was once in man a true happiness, of which all that now remains is the empty print and trace? This he tries in vain to fill with everything around him, seeking in things that are not there the help he cannot find in those that are, though none can help, since this infinite abyss can be filled only with an infinite and immutable object; in other words by God himself." In this he describes the search that is familiar to the fat girl. So many people are on this journey to fill that hole in their hearts.

Another time I met a beautiful young woman with an incredible singing talent. She is tall and blonde and beautiful in spite of the more than 100 pounds she wants to lose. She shared with me that when she was in high school, her stepfather was murdered. Before that she had never had a weight problem, but that event threw her into such a depression that she could hardly get out of bed in the morning. Her grades suffered, and she had to drop out of school for a while. She began eating to comfort herself in her grief.

These people suffered a pain that pierced their hearts like a bullet and left a hole that couldn't be healed. They needed the Comforter to heal them, but instead they turned to food. Does this sound familiar? Have your fat-girl tendencies to heal yourself left you more depressed and burdened with extra weight? Have you suffered in a way that you feel no one can understand? Do you feel that there is no way out of the pain that plagues you day and night? It's time to become the fit girl.

What a Fit Girl Knows

Fit girls know that making the right nutrition choices and getting regular exercise are only half the battle. The real key to losing weight and keeping it off is in fighting a spiritual and mental battle. When I lost all the weight while on *The Biggest Loser*, I found that many issues from my past reappeared. When it was time for the fit girl to deal with her internal fears and let go of the crutches the fat girl held on to for dear life, I felt like a scared kid curled up in a corner in a fetal position. I had to give that scared little girl permission to rise up and be strong. Why?

Because fit girls are strong and are not afraid to face challenges, obstacles, or their fears. I had to show the fat girl what a fit girl is capable of.

As a fat girl, I focused on naming things I couldn't do. After I started losing weight, I was on a mission to prove the fat girl wrong. I climbed mountains, kayaked rivers, hiked the Grand Canyon, and endured physical challenges that I never thought I could face. Being able to witness my own strength for the first time in my life and overcome the impossible was just the beginning of my fit-girl transformation. Healing my heart on the inside would prove to be a bigger challenge than climbing the biggest mountain I could find, but it was only when my heart healed that I was able to find the fit girl.

You may be asking, "Who is the fit girl?" The fit girl is *you* when you discover that the hole on the inside of you is designed to be filled by God, your heavenly Father and the Creator of the universe. The fit girl is *you* when you realize that the compulsion to fill an internal void with food, alcohol, or other stuff is futile because only God can fill that place. The fit girl is *you* when you realize that you don't need to comfort yourself with anything but God because you know He loves you very much and wants nothing but the best for your life.

The Bible says that "faith is the substance of things hoped for, the evidence of things not seen" (see Hebrews 11:1 NKJV). Faith in God is the belief that He is the substance you need for the life you dream of but have yet to see. For the fit girl, a life worth dreaming about is one where she doesn't have to fill the empty places in her life with things outside of God when pressures get to her.

Remember how I said I would continue to learn this lesson? Well, when I was going through the process of losing weight, I faced different kinds of temptations to fill the void. My new alternatives to filling the void were worse than the food addiction.

For instance, as I got thinner, I was getting attention from men other than my husband. I hadn't experienced that kind of attention in years, and to be honest, I liked it. In fact, I liked it so much that I realized that even though I was a happily married woman, I still sought after male attention to prove that I was attractive. I liked it when other men thought I was pretty, and so I didn't discourage harmless flirtations. As you can imagine, my husband didn't find this behavior an acceptable replacement for my food cravings.

Before I knew it, I found myself switching from one addiction to another. I stopped caring about welcoming glances from men and started drinking red wine. That occasional one glass of wine quickly turned into two or three glasses a few nights a week. Obviously the fat girl wasn't just an outside issue but an issue of the heart. I had a heart problem, and I needed a healer.

So once again I turned to the Lord and asked Him to heal me and be my guide. I asked Him to fill me with His Holy Spirit and show me how to change my heart. I asked Him to reveal to me the keys to change my reactions to life and its challenges and pressures. It was then that God, once again, asked me to have faith in Him and trust Him with my life. He didn't want to be my acquaintance. He wanted to be my Lord. Thankfully, I said yes to that process. I haven't looked back since.

What about you? Have you noticed that your struggles are similar to mine? Do you have a hole in your heart that you are trying to fill up with addictive behaviors like compulsive shopping, drinking too much, or smoking cigarettes? Have you lost weight and found yourself holding on to things that have replaced a food addiction? What's your new drug of choice?

Often weight can be a security blanket to keep from having to deal with sensitive things going on in the heart, and uncovering those hurts can be a painful process. Know this: God loves you and wants you to be whole and fit. He wants to build a relationship with you so that you can allow Him to fill every part of your life. It's not enough to occasionally chat with Him through a prayer. God wants to be your partner and your friend. He wants to transform you from the inside out! He wants you to be a fit girl.

> For everything you have missed, you have gained something else, and for everything you gain, you lose something else. —Ralph Waldo Emerson

～♨ TRANSFORMATION TIPS ♨～

I want you to do something for me. Find a really quiet place and go there by yourself. I know this might be hard if you have little kids or a busy schedule, but carve out some time to sit in the quiet and set your daily routine aside for a while. This is important. (By the way, finding a few minutes alone to meditate and pray is a great thing to do at the end of each of these lessons.)

During this quiet time, pray and ask God to reveal some things that may be holding you back from being the fit girl He made you to be. He may bring things to your mind that you haven't thought about in years. You may have buried feelings, situations, or experiences you didn't want to deal with back then—things God wants you to uncover today. God can show you these things through dreams or even nightmares. Identify whatever comes to your mind and write them down in a journal.

Here is a list of questions that will help you with this process and show you some things that may be keeping the fit girl at bay. Take some time to meditate on these questions and pray about your answers. Ask God to speak into your heart.

1. What are my earliest childhood memories? Are they happy ones? Sad ones?

2. How have these memories shaped my life?

3. Are there people from my past who I need to forgive or ask to forgive me?

4. What role does God have in my life? Can I draw closer to Him?

5. In my relationships with others, does the way I act cause hurt feelings? Concerning myself, does my behavior cause harm or is it self-destructive?

These might be hard questions for you to think about, but it's what you have to do if you want to transform yourself into a fit girl. Finally, I want you to pray about each revelation and ask God to show you how to make changes in the areas that need some work. Trust that He will give you the strategies to heal the places that need healing.

Commit to having a closer relationship with God and listening more closely when He speaks to your heart. He may ask you to call someone and ask them to forgive you for being angry with them. He may tell you that you are going to have to end relationships in your life that are unhealthy. Whatever it is you feel He is leading you to do, do it. This is the beginning of the healing journey and finding the fit girl in you!

⌇⌇ Your Prayer ⌇⌇

Father, please help me realize that only You can fulfill me, and that I need only You to fill the empty spaces inside me. Help me turn away from the temptation to fill my empty spaces with anything else. I pray that You would give me the strength to continually make the choice to relinquish control of my life to You. In Jesus' name I pray. Amen.

Food Has Whatever Power You Give It

If the word has the potency to revive and make us free,
it has also the power to blind, imprison, and destroy.

—RALPH ELLISON

Since I turned ten years old, I've been on every diet known to man. I've done them all. I have eaten cabbage soup, taken pills, experienced cleanses, and spent weeks not eating carbs. You can probably relate. If the definition of insanity is doing the same thing over and over and expecting different results, then I guess I was pretty crazy to expect diets to magically cure me from being fat. They never did. I never saw lasting results. When I became a fit girl, I finally realized diets are not the answer. They simply don't work.

Changing our eating habits for life is the only real way to become the fit girl we all desire to be. It is true, however, that what we eat has a major role in weight loss. We have to eat the right foods to fuel our bodies, and we have to use portion control to maintain a healthy weight.

Briefly, here are the practical golden rules of weight loss. These are truly important to being healthy because to lose weight, there are natural things you have to do to make it happen. You may have heard about them already, and you may even know them by heart. If so, that is great! Keep these things in your mind when we later combine them with the spiritual aspect of weight loss.

First of all, you have to drink water. Our bodies need water to function properly. How much water should you have? The rule of thumb that I have adopted is to take my body weight, divide it in half, and drink that much water in ounces. For example, if you weigh 150 pounds, you need to drink 75 ounces of water per day. Did you know that your body can actually hold on to weight if you are not properly hydrated? It's true. Drinking enough water is very important.

Secondly, keep track of your caloric intake. Many people don't have any idea how many calories they are eating each day. Although many eat too much, did you know it is possible to gain weight from eating too few calories? When someone diets and restricts their calories too much, their metabolism can actually slow down to the point that they are able to gain weight. I have found it helpful to have a notebook in my purse along with a calorie-counter book, so I can jot down the foods I eat and the calories in them. After a while remembering what you ate and counting those calories may become second nature to you, and you may not need to write them down. But, at least initially, it is a good idea to keep that list to hold you accountable.

If you are wondering what your calorie range should be, there are several online resources that can help you to determine that. I like the website dailyplate.com. On this website they have a place to type in your age, height, weight, and weight-loss goal. Once done, it will calculate the range of calories you should stay within to achieve your goal. That same website has a database of thousands of foods and their nutritional content. Instead of writing down what you eat, you can go to this site, input what you eat, and let it track the calories for you.

The third crucial rule is eat breakfast. Before I lost weight, I knew that it was important to watch calories, and so I would try to save them up until I was hungry. I tried to be good, and that meant I wouldn't eat. I was never hungry first thing in the morning, so I always skipped breakfast. Then by two o'clock, I was so ravenous I would grab the first thing I could find, and it was usually fast food. I went from one extreme to the other. I never felt those slight hunger pangs, which are a sign that you need to give your body a little fuel. I only got the emergency starvation pangs, which meant that my body was in starvation mode. What I didn't realize was that by skipping breakfast, I was actually training my metabolism to slow down. What I didn't know was that if I started the day off with a good breakfast, then I would actually jump-start my metabolism and set myself on a pattern to keep it cranking all day. Now I am always hungry in the morning, and that is a good sign. If you actually feel hungry, that means your metabolism is working. If you go for long periods through the day without feeling hungry and then suddenly feel ravenous, that may be a sign that your metabolism isn't working properly.

In addition, try to eat smaller meals, but eat them more often. For example, I get up in the morning and eat about 250 to 300 calories for breakfast. I usually eat two to three egg whites, a piece of wheat toast, and a slice or two of turkey bacon. Three to four hours later, I eat a snack. This could be a carton of Greek yogurt with a few almonds, which is about 200 calories, or a banana with some almond or peanut butter, also about 200 calories. I have lunch three or four hours later, then a snack, and then dinner. I am constantly putting wood on the fire to feed my metabolism, and at the same time, I'm being mindful of the calories.

This brings me to my next point. The way you combine your food is also very important. A balanced meal always includes protein, carbohydrates, and a little healthy fat. Previously, I told you that for breakfast I usually eat egg whites, turkey bacon (both are protein), and wheat toast (carbohydrates), and I cook them in olive oil cooking spray (healthy fat). The same thing applies to each snack. I had Greek yogurt (protein and carbohydrates) and almonds (healthy fat). It's important to combine your foods this way because carbohydrates give you energy while the protein helps to sustain that energy. This stabilizes your blood sugar so that you don't have to experience those spikes (highs) and crashes (lows). Remember when I told you that I would go most of the day without eating and then suddenly eat anything I could find? Well, after I ate, I had energy for only a short time. Before I knew it, I crashed. I felt so sleepy that I could barely function. This usually happened around the time my kids got home from school and needed me the most. Now I eat smaller meals with the proper macronutrient combinations, and this keeps my energy level stable all day.

It is also important to avoid white foods. These are foods like sugar, white flour, white pasta, and white rice. These foods have been stripped of the nutrients your body needs to function properly. I am particularly sensitive to sugar. If I eat foods that are loaded with sugar or high fructose corn syrup, I find that I crash quickly. I need my energy so I can't afford to let that happen.

We also need to look at our bodies as a place where God lives. We don't want to invite God into a shack. We want to give our bodies the things that will make them function as well as possible. Whole-wheat breads, whole-grain pastas, and foods that are less processed and relatively free of chemicals and sugar are simply better for our "temples."

Finally, watch your sodium. Recently, the Institute of Medicine, part of the National Academy of Sciences, issued a report that lowered the recommended daily amount of sodium. Previously, the daily allowance was 2500 milligrams, but it has been lowered to 1500 milligrams per day. As Americans we get so much extra sodium in the foods we eat—even in foods we might not expect to contain much sodium like cereals, ketchup, and cheese. Frozen meals, soups, and fast foods often have higher than the recommended daily allowance in just two servings!

Here is a list of some foods and their sodium content. Some of them may surprise you.

- Cheerios (1 cup): 190 milligrams
- 2 percent milk (8 ounces): 100 milligrams
- Starbucks Mocha Frappuccino: 160 milligrams
- Coke (12 ounce can): 49 milligrams
- McDonalds Big Mac: 1040 milligrams
- McDonalds French fries (medium): 221 milligrams
- Ketchup (4 packets): 440 milligrams

- Tombstone Original Pepperoni Pizza (¼ of a 12-inch frozen pizza): 880 milligrams
- Parmesan cheese (1 teaspoon): 76 milligrams
- Hostess CupCake (cream-filled): 290 milligrams

So just why is sodium so bad for us? Although we need it to keep the correct balance of fluid in our bodies, transmit nerve impulses, and aid in the contraction and relaxation of muscles, if we consume too much, the result is health problems. If we eat too much of it, the kidneys can't get rid of it through urination, so it then collects in the blood. This increases the volume of the blood and makes the heart have to work harder to pump the blood through the body. The result is high blood pressure. This, in turn, increases the chances of developing heart disease or having a stroke. Eating too much salt also causes the body to retain excess water and makes a person feel bloated. I rarely put extra salt on my food, but when I do, I use a salt substitute, which is actually potassium. By doing this I can prevent having excess sodium in my diet.

7 Golden Rules of Weight Loss

1. Drink water.
2. Keep track of your caloric intake.
3. Always eat breakfast.
4. Eat small meals every three to four hours.
5. Combine protein, carbohydrates, and healthy fat with every meal and snack.
6. Avoid white foods as much as possible.
7. Watch your sodium intake.

The biggest struggle to losing weight is not just the sweet (or salty) indulgences we can't seem to give up. It's about more than food. It's about our lack of control over food. It's about us allowing food to overpower us. It's what makes women say, "I just can't give up my soda first thing in the morning," or "I have a sweet tooth that I just can't get rid of."

Make no mistake. We need food to live. We need to eat to make enough energy for our bodies to work properly. But food does not need to be our master. We should only have one master, and that is God.

What You Say Matters

Now that we have talked about the practical things, I want to talk about your words. You can vow to do all the things I've written about and at the same time be sabotaging your efforts with what you say. Here's a little secret. When you say things about your lack of control over certain foods, you are practically admitting defeat before you even begin to wage war on the battle of the bulge. The Bible tells us, "For whatever is in your heart determines what you say" (Matthew 12:34 NLT). What you really believe in your heart is what will come out of your mouth!

> Nothing would be more tiresome than eating and drinking if God had not made them a pleasure as well as a necessity. —Voltaire

You learn what someone really believes when they talk about it all the time. The fat girl who says, "I just can't give up ice cream, candy, cake, and [fill in the blank]" is the woman who believes she is doomed by her unhealthy habits. Fat girls don't realize that they are their own worst enemies by proclaiming that food is more powerful than they are. They have made a personal prison with their own words.

On the journey to becoming the fit girl, we have to realize that we have power over food. Food seems to gain power only when we give over to it with our words and with our actions. Think about this. Do you really believe that a cookie is more powerful than you are? Of course not! So why do you say things like, "If it wasn't for my love of cookies, I would be ten pounds thinner." It's a ridiculous thought, isn't it? But if you say it out loud, you probably believe it in your heart.

I want to show you the connection between the fit girl and the power of her words. This truth is how we came into existence. In the Bible, the story of life is told in the book of Genesis. The story starts with God creating the world with His words. He said, "Let there be light," and there was light. He said, "Let there be trees, animals, and water," and they all came to be.

In different parts of the Bible, it also talks about how powerful our words are. I particularly like the third chapter of James. "When we put bits into the mouths of horses to make them obey us, we can turn the whole animal. Or take ships as an example. Although they are so large and are driven by strong winds, they are steered by a very small rudder wherever the pilot wants to go. Likewise the tongue is a small part of the body, but it makes great boasts. Consider what a great forest is set on fire by a small spark. The tongue also is a fire, a world of evil among the parts of the body. It corrupts the whole person, sets the whole course of his life on fire, and is itself set on fire by hell" (James 3:3-6).

Change Your Mind

Can you see the importance of what we talk about? The words that we say identify the beliefs that are in our heart. They speak of who we are in the very core of our being. Since I believe weight loss is as much a heart issue as it is a head issue, I believe that it is vital that we know the strategies to change fat-girl beliefs to fit-girl beliefs.

The first step to doing this is to transform our minds, so that what comes out of our mouths brings light, life, and truth. "Yes, I can get healthier." "No, I don't have to eat that cookie." "Yes, I can spend an hour today exercising." You may be thinking, *Amy, this sounds great, and maybe you're right, but how on earth can I possibly change my beliefs when it comes to food?*

Let me show you what the Bible has to say about this. In one of my favorite verses, this is what Jesus said. "I tell you the truth, if anyone says to this mountain, 'Go, throw yourself into the sea,' and does not doubt in his heart but believes that what he says will happen, it will be done for him. Therefore I tell you, whatever you ask for in prayer, believe that you have received it, and it will be yours" (Mark 11:23-24).

Spend a few minutes thinking about these verses. "Anyone" means you. Jesus is saying that *you* can ask for anything in prayer. This invitation is not reserved for super spiritual people, skinny people, or anyone you think is better than you for whatever reason.

Use Your Words

Here's another truth from this passage. Jesus wants us to talk to our mountain. This reminds me of when we were working with our son Rhett on his language skills. His autism made it difficult for him to ask for the things he wanted, but we had to teach him to ask. We repeatedly told him, "Use your words, Rhett." I think sometimes God is telling us the same thing. He is telling us to use our words when it comes to moving the mountains in our lives.

> If you wish to know the mind of a man, listen to his
> words. —Chinese Proverb

Think about the mountains in your life. What are they? Your addiction to sugar? A lack of time? A job crisis? What is standing in the way of you gaining health? Whatever it is, tell it to move! Tell it to get out of your way! Follow the example in the Bible and cast the mountain into the sea. Send it away so it never comes back. I assure you, when you say these things to your mountain and believe in your heart what you are saying, it will happen.

You need to start believing that the obstacle that is holding you back from the life you want to live can be cast away for good. Hebrews 11:6 tells us that "without faith it is impossible to please God." God wants you to trust Him to help in every area of your life. Philippians 4:13 (NKJV) says, "I can do all things through Christ who strengthens me." Don't you think God can give you strength to overcome the power food has in your life? Isn't He big enough to handle that challenge? If He created the whole world and knows the number of hairs on your head, I'm pretty confident He can handle whatever mountain is standing in your way.

I believe if you change your words about food based on Jesus' promise to us in Mark 11, your life can be different. I like to think of it as changing the tapes. If you are old enough to know what cassette tapes are, then you remember how popular it was for people to record a mix of their favorite songs. When they got tired of those songs, they could just record over them and make a new mix of songs.

It's the same principle when it comes to our minds replaying our beliefs about food. We may believe things about food that are destructive and, thus, live under the power of food. But remember, we can always record over those thoughts. We can tape a new mix of beliefs that are healthy.

I like to think that the fat girl dances to one kind of music and the fit girl to another. Their taped mixes are very different. The fat girl says, "I can't live without my bag of candy in the afternoon." The fit girl says, "I love water because it makes me feel so good, and it makes my body run properly." The fat girl says, "I'm hungry all the time. I can never get full." The fit girl says, "I have eaten a healthy meal, and I am satisfied." Do you see how just a few simple changes to what you say can make a huge difference? Try it out for yourself for a few days and see what happens.

Sometimes You Just Have to Fake It

When I started my journey to become a fit girl, a lot of fat-girl thinking had to change. I was painfully addicted to cheese and anything chocolate. I could not imagine eating pasta without smothering it in cheese or finishing a meal without enjoying a chocolate treat. I would say things like, "I don't like to have a salty taste in my mouth after I eat a meal, so I have to end my meals with something sweet."

During my transformation, I realized that I was so addicted to these two things that I abstained from them for a period of time. But more importantly, I had to retrain my brain to like healthier foods more than cheese and chocolate. Now, this didn't happen overnight. No food addict in their right mind is going to initially prefer broiled fish and steamed vegetables over cheesy pasta and chocolate. It takes time. And sometimes the only way you will really believe it is if you say it enough times. In my case, I told myself over and over that I liked broiled fish more than cheese. Yes, that's right. I actually said out loud, "I love this tilapia, asparagus, and sweet potato. Yum!" At first did I love it as much as I said I did? Of course not! But let me tell you what happened.

I found that after changing my eating habits for the better, my taste buds eventually changed, and I felt so much more energetic. I put two and two together and finally started believing the words that I was saying in my heart! My mind and heart lined up, and that connection created a new world of belief for me.

I am sure you have heard the saying, "If you tell yourself a lie long enough, you will begin to believe it." This is certainly true when it comes to changing the way you think about food (or anything for that matter). Talk to yourself and tell yourself what you like, even if it doesn't seem true at the time. This is the essence of faith; believing that the things you say will happen.

Don't let food control your life. Take charge over it. Take its power away. Proverbs 18:20-21 (NASB) says, "With the fruit of a man's mouth his stomach will be satisfied; he will be satisfied with the product of his lips. Death and life are in the power of the tongue, and those who love it will eat its fruit." We can choose to be healthy or not based on what we say and what we think. We have that power because Jesus died for us, and we can do "all things" through faith in His power working through us (see Philippians 4:13).

The Mind Is a Battlefield

The hardest fight a fat girl has to go through to become a fit girl is the battle of the mind or the thought life. Most of us have a countless number of thoughts entering our minds every day. Have you ever found yourself in the middle of doing something—such as watching TV, doing dishes, or talking to a friend—when suddenly you begin to think about the secret stash of cookies you hid on the top shelf in the pantry?

You know what I'm talking about. Those cookies are your favorite kind of chewy, gooey, lip-smacking, delicious chocolate-chip cookies. When the image of those treats enters your mind, you have some choices. You can either continue to think about those cookies, or you can think about something else. The cookies do not have to overpower your mind.

I heard a preacher once say that you can let a bird fly over your head, but you don't have to let it build a nest in your hair. We all have thoughts that come to us from time to time—we can't help it—but we have the power to choose whether or not to obsess over them or put them out of mind.

Here's an example. At one time or another, we have all been angry with someone. This doesn't make us a bad person. While you may want to slap someone who treated you unkindly, you know you won't do it (at least I hope not) because if you do, you'll likely suffer some consequences like getting arrested. So what do you do? You try to get over it. You make yourself stop harboring vindictive or harmful thoughts and feelings about this person. There is a big difference in thinking these things and acting them out.

It's the same thing with food. Most of us are used to obsessing over the cookie, the cake, the pasta, or whatever else catches our fancy. We visualize whatever it is that tempts us and before we know it, the thought turns into action, and we find ourselves actually eating what we were thinking about. We don't stop that bird from building a nest in our hair. In fact, we let it build a nest and lay some eggs.

In 2 Corinthians, the apostle Paul talks about the power that we have through God to cast thoughts that aren't good out of our minds. "The weapons we fight with are not the weapons of the world. On the contrary, they have divine power to demolish strongholds. We demolish arguments and every pretension that sets itself up against the knowledge of God, and we take captive every thought to make it obedient to Christ" (2 Corinthians 10:4-5).

Through Jesus, God has equipped us with weapons that are capable of casting out unhealthy thoughts that run rampant in our mind. When we are struck by a thought that can serve to sabotage or hurt us, we can redirect our thoughts. I know this is hard to do.

Let's go back to the chocolate-chip cookie example. (By the way, if you're not a cookie girl, you can imagine another kind of food you have a weakness for.) When you start thinking about the cookies, what does your mind start telling you? It starts telling you how good they would taste and how much better they would make you feel. It starts telling you that one cookie won't hurt. It starts telling you that you would be happy with just one bite. Before you know it, you are fixated on that cookie. Having a cookie becomes an obsession. All you can think about is the cookie. The cookie is controlling your mind, your emotions, your feelings, and your actions.

The cookie actually becomes a stronghold. This is when you have made up your mind that you have got to have that cookie! Wild horses couldn't stop you from running to the pantry and getting it. This is why it is so important to stop your want for a cookie (or anything else you are craving) when it is in the thought stage.

One strategy to help you win the battle of the mind is to distract yourself. When I start obsessing about a particular food and my mind is trying to convince me I've *got* to have it, I've found it helpful to distract myself with another thought or activity. For example, if I am home at night and I start having thoughts about cheese-smothered pizza, I'll go do something else. If I'm watching television, I may take a bath or do housework. Changing locations can usually jar me out of a destructive thought pattern and on to better thoughts.

I also notice that I've got triggers. Sometimes being in a certain place can remind me of old habits, and I can easily find myself back in the food-obsessed thought pattern. I often experience a lot of temptation to eat things I shouldn't when I am relaxing on the sofa at night. For me snacking while watching television became a habit through the years, so sometimes I still associate the couch and nighttime with snacking. This is my trigger.

You might have a different trigger. It may be hard for you to go to family barbeques because your family has a habit of eating all day until they can't eat anymore. Maybe going to the movies is your down-fall because watching a movie without eating popcorn and candy just doesn't seem normal. Whatever your particular weakness, realize that they might trigger harmful food-obsessed thoughts at any time. Be on guard. Shift gears. Do something else. Distract yourself.

Fit girls know that their words and thoughts ultimately create the life they want. When I started my health journey as the fat girl, I was in a prison that I had created for myself. My body and self-esteem sagged under the weight of extra pounds, wrong beliefs, and bad choices I had made. Though at first I felt hopeless about battling it out with my mind and transforming my beliefs, day by day I started to see more hope, change, and growth. It was a hard battle, but I was determined it was mine to win.

The more I practiced choosing what I say and changing my thought patterns, the stronger I became. During this process, something else happened. The fat girl got weaker and weaker, until one day she disappeared!

Don't get me wrong. In the battlefield of my mind, there are times when fat-girl thoughts fly over my head. The fit girl in me has learned how to recognize them for what they are—merely thoughts. The fit girl immediately casts them out of her head and moves on, knowing that those thoughts no longer control her.

Find a Friend

Having an accountability partner is another thing that has helped me control the way I see food. For me, it's Phillip. Some days I will tell him, "I have already eaten my limit for the day, so please don't let me eat anything else." This confession makes it more difficult for me to go into the kitchen and eat something that I shouldn't. Because I verbally asked for his help, I feel more responsible to keep my word and watch my eating habits.

Phillip does his job, though, too. Sometimes he will nag me and watch me like a hawk, usually until I just give up even thinking about eating something else. I'm proud of him because this is quite a change from the old Phillip. In the past, my husband wouldn't have been my best choice for an accountability partner. He used to be my enabler and brought home ice cream to me every night.

This brings me to an important lesson I've learned since I became a fit girl. Many times the people you are the closest to can sabotage your efforts to become healthy. They may intend to show their love for you by giving you treats like candy or making a special recipe for you. As kindhearted as they may be, this is not love. They are only hindering your efforts. You must be firm when it comes to being responsible for your health goals and not sabotage them by making someone happy by eating.

It's not uncommon for a person to work toward becoming healthy without the support of their spouse. If you are in this type of situation, look elsewhere for an accountability partner. Ask a friend, a neighbor, or a coworker.

One of the best ways to keep your mind in check during your transformation into a fit girl is to surround yourself with people who love you, support you, and root for your success. This is vital for you to reach your goals. I've been blessed to have a lot of friends who help me control myself when it comes to food, especially when I'm out at parties or other social events. My friend Phebe is one of my accountability partners. When we go out to a social function, we make sure we don't allow each other to fall into temptation.

Choosing different accountability friends for different settings is a good idea. While Phebe is great to have around me at parties, I've learned the benefits of having a group-support system. When I was on my weight-loss journey, I leaned on many different people who had different roles and influenced me for the better. I had the support of nutrition experts who helped me with my diet. I had gym buddies who helped me with my workouts. I had friends I went walking with and friends with whom my husband and I cooked healthy dinners. Our friends Tim and Carol are a wonderful couple. We love to go to dinner with them because they understand and share our healthy mind-set. When we are together, we are always guaranteed good times and healthy food.

Take a look around and see who you can use to build up your support system. Maybe your sister would like to become your walking partner. Maybe your mother wants to help you with choosing the right foods. Maybe your friend at church would like to pray for you. Whoever you choose to include in your health journey, be sure they support you and your goals. You'll be surprised at how many people you will find to help you along your way. I'm sure there are plenty of folks in your life who want to cheer you on and see you succeed.

Fit Girls Know How to Run

I like to read Hebrews 11 when I need to put the battle with food into perspective. This chapter recounts all the great things that men and women just like you and me were able to do through their faith in God. You can find the definition of faith in the beginning of the chapter, and then the text jumps into what many call the "faith hall of fame." The writer talks about Bible legends like Abraham, Joseph, and Moses and chronicles the amazing things they were able to do by faith. These men and women believed God was more powerful than any obstacle they faced.

Abraham believed that he would be the father of many nations even though he and his wife were too old to have children. Moses believed God could do great things for the people of Israel, even though he was growing up in an Egyptian palace. The people of Jericho believed God could bring down the walls of the city when they marched around them for seven days. It's encouraging and empowering to read this text.

I love the next chapter even more. "Therefore, since we are surrounded by such a great cloud of witnesses, let us throw off everything that hinders and the sin that so easily entangles, and let us run with perseverance the race marked out for us. Let us fix our eyes on Jesus, the author and perfecter of our faith, who for the joy set before him endured the cross, scorning its shame, and sat down at the right hand of the throne of God. Consider him who endured such opposition from sinful men, so that you will not grow weary and lose heart" (Hebrews 12:1-3).

The "great cloud of witnesses" refers to the great men and women of faith who were described in the previous chapter. I like to think that there is a stadium in heaven filled with all of these saints who have gone before us. I also believe that our Christian relatives who have passed away are there. I like to think about my grandfather, a Pentecostal preacher, sitting up in the stands of heaven, looking down at me, and grinning. I like to think that my great-grandmother, who taught me Bible verses as a child, is also sitting in the stands. Maybe she is even sitting next to Mary, the mother of Jesus, or Mother Teresa.

I like to imagine that every time I trust God in a time of temptation or in a difficult situation, they all stand up and cheer for me. As I patiently run my race and continue my journey, like the writer of Hebrews talks about, I have my own cheerleading section in heaven rooting for me.

Living life is like being in a race. We are running to win. I am running to beat my food addiction. You are running to overcome your own food issues. As a fat girl, you start running this race with a little bit of faith. But as you keep running, your faith builds up, and you start to use it more and more to overcome temptations. You run the race, build your faith, and start changing the words that come out of your mouth. You run the race, build your faith, and start controlling the thoughts that you allow to stay in your mind. You run the race, build your faith, and begin to "throw off everything that hinders" you.

Before you know it, the fit girl emerges, and the cloud of witnesses in your life begins to cheer. See, anytime you trust God to help you overcome an obstacle that is holding you back, you are pleasing Him (and that pleases your personal cheerleaders in heaven).

Where are you in your race? If you are starting that race as the fat girl, it's okay; keep running. Are you in the middle and feeling discouraged? It's okay; keep running. Are you near the finish line and getting a little tired? It's okay; keep running.

Your Turn

Right now I want you to think about the relationship you have with food. Have you struggled with certain eating patterns and habits and feel they are stronger than your will to fight them? Do you have core beliefs that you have held onto like a security blanket and don't feel capable of letting go? Are there certain times when you know your will to fight off cravings will be weaker than others? Do thoughts of weakness plague you during these times and tempt you to give in?

I know what you are going through. I have been there. You are in a battle to defeat the fat girl. But guess what? The fit girl is ready, willing, and able to win that battle, and she is right there inside of you! Not only that, but God wants to get involved in the process.

You might say to yourself, *Why would God care about helping me with my weight?* Let me tell you why. When you are fit and healthy, you are taking care of the creation God made. When you are taking care of yourself, you are able to fulfill the purpose God specifically created you for. When you are fulfilling His purpose, you are able to bless other people. Being a fit girl is a big deal to God! In 3 John 1:2 (NKJV), John tells us, "Beloved I pray that you may prosper in all things and be in health, just as your soul prospers." Our health is important to God. He wants to help you in your fight against the fat girl.

⸙ TRANSFORMATION TIPS ⸙

Now is your moment of decision. This is your moment of reckoning. Are you going to make the changes necessary to transform into the fit girl? If so, this is what you need to do. You need to watch the words that come out of your mouth regarding your habits with food. Once you identify those negative words you've been in the habit of saying, you need to turn them around. Replace those words, and ultimately beliefs, with more positive and healthy ones. Make this a new reality in your life.

You also need to learn to deal with the destructive thoughts that pass through your mind before they become imaginations and ultimately strongholds. Just because you ride by an ice-cream parlor and think about ice cream doesn't mean you have to keep thinking about it until you have to eat a scoop or two. You have the power in you through God to distract yourself and keep driving. I believe in you, and I know that as you read this book, you'll become the fit girl.

1. Write down all the thoughts that come into your mind for one day. Can you identify anything you are saying that could sabotage your weight-loss goals? Write down what you've identified.

2. Write down positive affirmations you can substitute for negative thoughts. For example, if you think you can't give up candy, remind yourself that you can do all things through Jesus Christ. If you think you can't eat healthier, tell yourself that you deserve to put the right foods into your body to make it

work the way God designed it to work. Practice saying those new positive statements to yourself daily. Notice how these new, positive words become true for you.

3. Think of ways you can distract yourself from overwhelming thoughts about food. Perhaps you'll choose to take a brisk walk, read the Bible, or call a friend. Find ways to divert your attention so when you start battling in your mind, you have a strategy to defeat the negative thoughts.

4. Find two people you can rely on as accountability partners. Talk to them about helping you with your journey. See how they can influence your life in a positive way and help you make and maintain the right changes in your life.

Your Prayer

Father, I trust that You are helping me replace my destructive thought patterns with new and healthy ones. I believe that through Christ I can do all things. I believe that You are all powerful, and that food no longer has power over me. I cast down all thoughts that can take me off my path to health. I throw off everything that hinders me from running the race You have set before me. I give my life to You and honor You by taking care of my temple. In Jesus' name I pray. Amen.

Your Thoughts

Rocky Road Is Not
Your Boyfriend's Name

Forget love, I'd rather fall in chocolate.

—Author Unknown

When I was a teenager, I wrote out an extensive and detailed list of all the things I wanted in a husband, my future life partner. I prayed over that list almost every day for a long time. I listed the obvious qualities like a good sense of humor and a cute smile, but I also wrote down some things that might have seemed a little strange to some people. If you read the list, you might have even thought I was nuts.

For instance, I wanted my husband to carry peppermints in his pockets so that when he was a grandfather, his grandkids would always know that their grandpa had candy to give them. I don't know what my thought process was to come up with that detail. I guess I wanted him to be like a Santa Claus figure to his grandchildren.

The one thing I knew for sure was that I wanted to get married. I wanted to meet someone I could share my life with. I had a deep longing for that one person who I knew would walk through life with me. Now, I don't believe that everyone needs to get married or even that it is God's plan for everyone, but for me it was a very strong desire.

When I met my husband, Phillip, one of the first things he did was put his hand in his pocket and offer me a peppermint. My mouth dropped, and my heart skipped a beat. I took it as a sign that I needed to keep my eyes on this guy. Sure enough, we were married only a few years later, and as of this writing, we are not far away from celebrating our twenty-fifth wedding anniversary. I believe that God brought this relationship into my life to give me a partner I could help and who could support me.

Wired for Relationship

God created us as relational beings. He created us to desire a relationship with Him above all, but He also put in us the desire and need to maintain and nurture strong relationships with others. We all need family, friends, and mentors to support, strengthen, and encourage us in life. There is no substitute for those bonds.

Do you remember the movie *Jerry McGuire*? Do you remember when the main character, played by Tom Cruise, went through a long-winded speech with his love interest, Dorothy, who was played by Renee Zellweger, about how he felt about her? Most of us remember his famous last line, "You complete me." And, of course, most of us remember Dorothy's follow-up line, the one that Kenny Chesney wrote a song about, "You had me at hello."

Those of us who are die-hard romantics shed tears of joy during this scene. We were so happy for this young couple because in this great big world full of people, these two had found the person who was made for them. They found their "other."

As Christians, we know that no one person in this world can truly complete us other than God. But because we are wired to be in relationship with God and others, we need to share our lives with people. We need that connection. We need that bond. It is what helps to shape us into the people God has called us to be. Usually we are even transformed into better people because of the relationships that matter most to us—whether it's with your spouse, your best friend, your parents, or your sister. Think about this. Even Jesus had His disciples, some of His best buddies, who He shared His life with. And we're talking about the Son of God!

Don't we all want this? Don't we all want to have friends in our lives who love us no matter what? Don't we all want to have family who support us through the hard times and cheer us on during the happy ones?

The Fat Girl's Skewed View of Relationship

I've noticed that many times, the fat girl doesn't understand the importance of relationship. She might not even know what a good one looks like. I'm sure most of you dated someone who was a bad boy. You know the type. He's the guy who breaks your heart by telling you he loves you but then cheats on you. He is emotionally unavailable, and though you would do anything for him, he couldn't care less. He's the guy who is verbally or physically abusive. Sometimes we stay in bad relationships because we don't think we deserve better or we're afraid of being alone.

The fat girl may even be too afraid of being abandoned by people, so she simply runs away from or avoids intimacy at all costs. She may view relationships with others as an ultimately painful experience, so she substitutes that God-given need with something else. In the case of the fat girl, it's food.

When Food Becomes Your Friend

The odd thing is an unhealthy relationship with food can be worse than one of those relationships with a bad boy. Here is what you need to know about food addiction. Food has no conscience or emotion. Just like a little girl who talks to a stuffed animal and thinks that maybe it will magically come to life and be her friend, we sometimes mistakenly think that food can fill some kind of void in our lives because it means something other than helping our physical bodies survive. This is a fairy tale that will never come true.

Food may not be able to hurt you emotionally, but it can hurt you physically and keep you from fulfilling your dreams. Food doesn't care about you, how you feel, or what your future goals are. Food doesn't care whether or not you live or die. Food doesn't care whether or not your heart is broken or if you have had a victory in your life.

When we turn to food for comfort, we are destined to fall into a vicious cycle. Here's what I mean. When we overeat for comfort, we gain weight. When we gain weight, we become depressed, so we eat more to make ourselves feel better. The cycle continues, and we become more isolated from others because we become more self-conscious about how we look. This kind of relationship with food is unhealthy and unfulfilling.

You need to realize once and for all that food cannot take the place of healthy, solid relationships with people who can love and support you. Food cannot replace your relationship with God or those relationships that are ordained by God to fulfill you and make your life more joyful and meaningful.

This is something that the fit girl realizes. She understands that food is a tool that is meant to be used to fuel our bodies, not something that controls our behaviors, actions, and feelings. While the fat girl uses food to comfort herself, the fit girl turns to God and God-given relationships to provide comfort.

My Unhealthy Cycle

When I was the fat girl, I remember all too well how comfortable I became living in my own vicious cycle. I avoided contact with people and social situations as much as possible because I felt trapped inside a body and a mentality that weighed me down. Going places required a harrowing ritual of trying to find clothes that both fit and looked decent on me. If an outfit looked okay, I spent an hour doing my hair and makeup to complete my perfect look.

It took me forever just to get ready for work or leave the house for any reason. I didn't even go to Walmart at midnight without looking as perfect as I could, the extra pounds and all. In my mind, if my hair and makeup looked fabulous, then maybe no one would notice the extra hundred pounds on my body.

I constantly wondered if people were looking at me and what they were thinking. I hated looking at full-length mirrors, so I never kept any around the house. I was so self-conscious that it was exhausting! I would rather sit at home by myself, watch television, and snack than hang out with friends and be social. There were many times when I was out with my girlfriends and secretly wished that I was alone at home in my jammies with a bag of chips and a good movie.

That was when I knew that my relationship with food was definitely a problem. Its hold on me was so strong that I actually preferred to be in a relationship with food than with other people. But this was not how God created me to live.

Fit-Girl Cycles

When I became a fit girl, I suddenly realized how limiting my life had been. I had tried to stay in a comfortable little box for so long. The problem was that until I got out of it, I didn't realize how uncomfortable it had really become. I couldn't see how much my lifestyle—my unhealthy relationship with food—had prohibited me from really living life!

Suddenly, the world opened wide with possibilities. Things that I never even thought about doing before were suddenly possible—simple things like going dancing with my husband without being embarrassed or being able to find flattering clothes that accentuated my figure. These are things that most people take for granted. When you are living the life of a fat girl, you are confined to a box. When you live the life of a fit girl, the box disappears, and you are left with a bigger world.

When my world got bigger, I had so many places to go and people to meet. No longer held captive by the deadly grip of food, I was free to live the kind of life God intended for me to live. My relationship with food was no longer a priority because I had learned the true purpose of food—to fuel my body so it can function at an optimal level.

My Love Story

When I read the story of Adam and Eve in Genesis, I think about how the story is not only about the fall of man, but also a study in human relationships and a commentary on the way God made His creatures. In the beginning, God created the heaven and the earth, and then He created man, Adam. Shortly after that, God looked down, and even though Adam had full access to God, He recognized that Adam was still lonely. Even though Adam could engage in one-on-one time with his Lord whenever he wanted, a piece of Adam was still missing. God knew that, and that's why He said that it is not good for man to be alone.

I find that fascinating. Adam was walking and talking with God every day, and yet God referred to Adam as being alone. Can you relate? Have you ever been in a room full of people and, yet, felt alone? You might even be in a relationship with someone and feel alone. God knew that Adam needed genuine and healthy human companionship. While there is no doubt that our relationship with God has to be the most important thing in our lives, God recognizes our need to be with others. That is why God took a rib out of Adam and created Eve. Notice that when God said it wasn't good for man to be alone, He didn't create ice cream or pizza. He created Eve.

I know a little bit about how Adam must have felt. Phillip and I started dating in college, and after a few months, we broke up. Even though I felt like he was "the one," apparently the feeling wasn't mutual. I was very lonely after he called our relationship off. Shortly after that, he decided to go into the United States Air Force, and I lost touch with him. During this time, I made a decision to get closer to God and try to figure out what He wanted for my life. Whatever it was, I was going to do it.

I spent a couple of years going to school and helping out at my church. While praying for my future, I decided that I should enroll in classes at a Bible college in Oklahoma and begin training for the ministry the next semester. For some reason, I started thinking about Phillip. I hadn't talked to him in over two years and found myself wondering about what was happening in his life. I assumed that he was still in the air force and based in California.

One day I had a feeling I should call him. It was weird. I didn't know why the feeling was so strong. Maybe I was supposed to minister to him and tell him about my deepening relationship with God. I called his mother to get his number, and to my surprise, I learned that Phillip was not in California, but in Oklahoma. He was actually attending the same college I had applied to!

I had this odd feeling that God was up to something. I called Phillip, and his roommate, Dan, answered the phone. When he yelled for Phillip to pick up the other line, he said, "Your wife's on the phone." I was struck again by a powerful feeling. Was this some sort of sign?

Phillip and I talked for hours. We caught each other up on what was going on in our lives, and he even told me that he had decided Jesus was his "girlfriend" for the time being. It may seem like a strange thing to say, but it assured me that he was devoted to God, and I definitely appreciated that commitment. Phillip continued to call me once a week. The more we talked, the more I fell in love with him all over again.

A couple of months later, Phillip called to tell me he was coming home to visit and wanted to get together. We went to church the first night after our reunion. The following evening he asked if I wanted to watch a movie with him at his parents' house. I went over there and couldn't help staring at him all googly-eyed. I was so smitten. I tried not to let my feelings show because clearly he wasn't sending any googly eyes my way. Two days later, he called, and with a trembling voice, he asked me if we could meet. I agreed, and we met at the mall.

We walked around for hours, and I still had no idea why he had called this meeting. We had even had our picture taken with the Easter Bunny and driven around downtown in the car. Phillip hadn't said anything that indicated why it was so urgent that he see me. A few hours later, he started looking a little uncomfortable. He said (and I quote), "Has God been saying anything to you about me?" What a loaded question! Here I was in love with the guy and counting the signs on my hand why I believed he was the one for me. I said yes, and we continued to talk about it. Finally he told me, "I feel like you are supposed to be my wife."

So I did what any good Southern woman would do. I told him to get down on his knees and ask me to marry him. He did and I said yes (even though a really good Southern woman wouldn't say yes until she had also been presented with a diamond ring—but he took care of that later on). We were married six months later.

I tell you that story to emphasize that God cares about our relationships and brings people together in miraculous ways. What if I didn't follow my heart and call Phillip that day to see what he was doing? I could have sat at home, stuffed my face, and felt sorry for myself, and I would have never found the love of my life.

There is no substitute for the relationships God brings into your life. Food cannot be your boyfriend or girlfriend. Food cannot even be your friend. Turning to it for comfort, acceptance, love, respect, or to feel warm and fuzzy will never satisfy the longings of your heart that are intended for a relationship with God and others.

Time to Break Up with Food

What about you? Do you think that Rocky Road is the name of your boyfriend, and are you having a love affair with ice cream? It could be something else. What food are you having a secret rendezvous with? What food do you hide and eat when no one is looking? It may be a favorite junk food, but it also may be a healthy food that you are eating too much of. It can be any kind of food that gives you an emotional release from a stressful day. Are you using food to soothe yourself? Are you using food as a coping mechanism to deal with life?

If so, these are indications that you may need to re-evaluate your relationship with food. Food can be as addictive as any drug and more so because we have to eat to survive. You can stop drinking alcohol forever, but you can't quit eating. This makes fighting a food addiction more difficult, but be encouraged. It's definitely possible to let go of that addiction.

There is hope that you can change the way you think about food and your relationship with it. You can break up with your food of choice today. I'm going to show you ways to change your unhealthy thought process toward food so that you can become a fit girl!

What Your Relationship with Food Shouldn't Look Like

Let me be clear on this point. Food is not your friend, family, or boyfriend. Food cannot bring you comfort or fill the holes in your soul. So why do we turn to it when we are sad or feel emotional? Why do we let it rule our lives to the point that we aren't living the best life we can live? Why do we let it rob us of self-confidence because of the excess weight it brings to our bodies?

Are You a Food Addict?

To answer this question, ask yourself the following questions, which are found on the Food Addicts Anonymous in Recovery website (www.foodaddicts.org), and answer them as honestly as you can.

1. Have you ever wanted to stop eating and found you just couldn't?
2. Do you think about food or your weight constantly?
3. Do you find yourself attempting one diet or food plan after another, with no lasting success?
4. Do you binge and then "get rid of the binge" through vomiting, exercise, laxatives, or other forms of purging?
5. Do you eat differently in private than you do in front of other people?
6. Has a doctor or family member ever approached you with concern about your eating habits or weight?
7. Do you eat large quantities of food at one time (binge)?
8. Is your weight problem due to your "nibbling" all day long?
9. Do you eat to escape from your feelings?
10. Do you eat when you're not hungry?
11. Have you ever discarded food, only to retrieve it and eat it later?
12. Do you eat in secret?
13. Do you fast or severely restrict your food intake?
14. Have you ever stolen other people's food?

15. Have you ever hidden food to make sure you have "enough"?

16. Do you feel driven to exercise excessively to control your weight?

17. Do you obsessively calculate the calories you've burned against the calories you've eaten?

18. Do you frequently feel guilty or ashamed about what you've eaten?

19. Are you waiting for your life to begin "when you lose the weight"?

20. Do you feel hopeless about your relationship with food?

If you answered yes to any of the above questions, then you may be a food addict.

When I was living with the fat girl, I looked at food a certain way. I saw some foods as good and others as bad. I tried to resist eating like you try to resist calling a guy you know is bad news. I starved myself all day, and then in the late afternoon, when I couldn't stand it anymore, I broke down and ate until I couldn't eat any more. Right before bedtime, I practically immersed myself in a bowl of ice cream because I figured I had ruined my diet for the day and might as well keep the trend going. I resolved to have more willpower the next day. The problem was the next day was pretty much the same.

What Your Relationship with Food Should Be

I will never forget the day that I found the fit girl. Someone told me that I needed to look at food the same way I look at putting gas in my car. In other words, I was to look at food as a way to fuel my body. This was a wonderful illustration for me because at the time I drove a gas-guzzling SUV that I had to constantly fill up with gas. I figured I couldn't drive on an empty tank all day, and so why should I go all day without putting food into my body? Of course, this went against the fat-girl mentality that you should try to eat as little as possible and starve yourself. No wonder I was hungry all the time!

I always knew that to lose weight, you have to burn more calories than you take in. As a fat girl, I remember thinking that I would not eat all day, save up those calories, and pig out at night. I thought it didn't matter as long as I stayed under a certain number of calories. Calories were calories. I figured it didn't matter if the calories came from an apple or a chocolate bar.

When I became a fit girl, everything changed. I realized I was tired all the time because I wasn't getting the right number of calories into my body, and the calories weren't coming from nutritious foods. I learned that a human being needs to be fueled often and in small amounts. I also needed to eat foods that were high in nutrients. Just as I wouldn't want to put water into my SUV gas tank, I wouldn't want to put junk or processed foods into my body. It wouldn't run efficiently.

Most of us don't know how to fuel our bodies. We don't know when to eat, how to eat, or what to eat. I told you before that this book is not a diet book. There are plenty books out there to teach you the fundamentals of nutrition, but there are basic food rules you can start learning today to help you see food as fuel and not as anything else.

In the last chapter, I wrote in detail about some practical eating tips. Go back and review those tips again. When you focus on these simple rules, you can help your body work properly and effectively. You will feel energized, look healthy, and have a better mental attitude. The fit girl keeps this good information at the forefront of her mind.

I cannot stress this enough—food cannot replace people. It cannot make you happy or soothe your heart when you are sad. What it can do for you—if you use it properly—is give you energy. If you make the right food choices, it can help you to be healthy and well. The fit girl knows a good relationship with food means better health.

Eating is not an emotional experience. It is a practical one. It's like brushing your teeth. The fit girl knows that eating is just another daily thing that has to be done in order for her to stay healthy and run her human "car" properly. When your body runs properly, the limits that once held you back come off, and the world becomes a bigger and more exciting place. You can see dreams you once gave up on become possible again. You stop being self-conscious and become more conscious of the blessings God has given you through the relationships He has placed into your life. All this wonderful change comes by just flipping the switch on the way you think about food.

> Strength is the ability to break a chocolate bar into four pieces with your bare hands—and then eat just one of those pieces. —Judith Viorst

⟨⟨⟨❧ TRANSFORMATION TIPS ❧⟩⟩⟩

You may be realizing that you have an unhealthy relationship with food. Many experts call this being an "emotional eater." I want to give you some useful suggestions to help you stop this destructive pattern and start thinking of food only as a way to fuel your body.

1. Examine the relationships in your life. Do you notice any particular patterns that keep repeating themselves? Do you find that you keep getting abused or abandoned? If so, pray and ask God to show you the root of this problem. Many times there is an event from your past that is so traumatic that you bury the memory by eating to comfort that pain. You may need a licensed therapist or support group to help you navigate through this process. Many churches have recovery groups that can help you deal with these issues.

2. Think about and write down your reactions to social invitations. If someone asks you to go on a date or your friends invite you to a party, do you secretly prefer to stay at home, watch a good television show, and eat snacks? If a friend asks you to go shopping, do you get nervous, self-conscious, and wish you could just go shop alone? If so, these may be

indications that you have become afraid of getting close to people. You may have been hurt by relationships and are too scared to put yourself back out there. If so, you need to start accepting some of those invitations and face that fear. The fear is always scarier than the reality. You might surprise yourself and have a great time when you start saying yes to social events!

3. Don't view the relationships in your life through the eyes of past hurts. If someone steps on your toe (figuratively speaking), the tendency is always to pull your foot back when they walk by again. If you are constantly expecting people to hurt you and let you down, then they probably will. The Bible tells us that whatever we think, we are (see Proverbs 23:7). Whatever you believe and expect is what will happen to you. Try to look at each relationship with a positive expectation.

4. Look at your relationships from the perspective of blessing the people God has brought into your life. The more you think about the needs of others, the less you think about yourself. If you are not so worried about yourself, then you are not looking for ways for people to hurt you. Instead, you are looking for ways that you can make other's lives better. When you give to another person, it always comes back to you.

5. Start looking at your past experiences with relationships as opportunities to learn. Maybe you were taken advantage of in a business deal, or maybe your best friend betrayed you in some way. These scenarios could make you want to harden your heart and not trust people in the future. Don't allow them to make you bitter but do allow them to make you better!

6. Look at the Food Addicts Anonymous Twelve Steps and see if there are some ideas you need to start practicing.

Food Addicts Anonymous Twelve Steps*

1. We admitted we were powerless over our food addiction—that our lives had become unmanageable.

2. Came to believe that a Power greater than ourselves could restore us to sanity.

3. Made a decision to turn our will and our lives over to the care of God as we understood God.

4. Made a searching and fearless moral inventory of ourselves.

5. Admitted to God, to ourselves, and to another human being the exact nature of our wrongs.

6. Were entirely ready to have God remove all these defects of character.

7. Humbly asked God to remove our shortcomings.

8. Made a list of all persons we had harmed and became willing to make amends to them all.

9. Made direct amends to such people wherever possible, except when to do so would injure them or others.

10. Continued to take personal inventory and when we were wrong promptly admitted it.

11. Sought through prayer and meditation to improve our conscious contact with God as we understood God, praying only for knowledge of God's will for us and the power to carry that out.

12. Having had a spiritual awakening as the result of these steps, we tried to carry this message to food addicts and to practice these principles in all our affairs.

*see www.foodaddictsanonymous.org/faas-twelve-steps

Will people let you down and hurt you sometimes? Of course! No one is perfect. But that should never stop us from pursuing and nurturing healthy relationships with others. When we focus more on maintaining good friendships, we will focus less on using food to substitute for others. We must embrace relationships with people so that we can have the fulfilling life that God intended for us to have!

⸎ Your Prayer ⸎

Father, I pray that You would fill my life with the relationships You have placed in my life on purpose. I pray You give me friends who can support me and help me make the necessary choices so that the fit girl can thrive. I pray that I would not be self-conscious or afraid but willing to reach out to other people and develop relationships that will make my life fuller. Thank You for helping me be accountable to others and to You. In Jesus' name I pray. Amen.

Your Thoughts

When Emotions Eat at You, Don't Eat Back!

Gluttony is an emotional escape, a
sign something is eating us.

—Peter De Vries

When I was about five years old, I remember going on one particular trip to the grocery store with my mom. While we were browsing in the produce department, I noticed these cute, little cherry tomatoes. They were so pretty and red and looked just the right size for me. Suddenly, this overwhelming desire to eat one of those tomatoes overtook me. I felt like Goldilocks wanting to eat the little bear's porridge.

When Mom wasn't looking, I grabbed one and popped it into my mouth. It only took a moment for her to realize that I had something in my mouth. Like most mothers, she freaked out. She probably thought I was eating used gum or something I had picked off the dirty floor. When I explained to her that I just wanted to eat one of the pretty tomatoes, she got really quiet, and a disappointed look came over her face.

She explained to me that it was not okay to take things that don't belong to me. It was called "stealing," and stealing is not good. Like Adam and Eve getting caught eating the forbidden fruit, in that moment I knew I had done something wrong. I was ashamed of myself, and for the first time, I came face-to-face with the emotion of guilt.

The Power of Emotions

God created us with a soul, which consists of our mind, will, and emotions. Therefore, we feel things like guilt, sadness, happiness, and fear. While we don't have control over an initial feeling, we can control how we manage our emotions. If we are angry, does the anger consume us? If we are happy, do we live in a happy bubble and forget about everyone around us? If we feel guilty, do we stop living life because our shame is paralyzing?

The difference between being a fit girl and a fat girl is how you deal with your emotions. Let's use guilt as an example. What are some things you have felt guilty about? Every one of us has been guilty of doing something we shouldn't have done. If we were perfect, Jesus wouldn't have needed to die on the cross for our sins. When you feel guilty, the feeling is there to motivate you to run to Him for forgiveness.

Have you ever had a friend betray you and afterward withdrew from you even after you forgave her? This is a common reaction to feelings of guilt. I can always tell when my children have done something they shouldn't have. They usually pull away from me and don't want to spend time with me. When I ask them a question, they give me a quick short answer and then escape to their rooms. They feel guilty!

My youngest son, Rhett, who is autistic, loves to eat. We have repeatedly tried to keep certain foods, like sweets, away from him. He especially loves foods that aren't healthy for him. When we don't keep sweets in the house, he turns to fruit or bread or anything that turns to sugar in his system. There was a time when Rhett would sneak food and take it up to his bedroom. When we noticed the food disappearing, we asked him about it. He became really quiet. When we investigated his room, we found banana peels, apple cores, and bread crumbs in different parts of his room. I even found dried-up banana peels in his nightstand drawer. Gross! That evidence solved the question of the disappearing food. We had our little culprit!

However, before we found the evidence, the way he had been pulling away from me was one sure sign that he was the one responsible. Don't we do the same thing? When we feel guilty because of something hurtful we have done to someone, don't we try to retreat from them and comfort ourselves? It is a form of escapism. Escapism is a way to shield ourselves from our present reality by escaping to some other activity. You can use things like reading, travelling, or going to movies to do this, or you can use food. Using food is the primary way the fat girl escapes.

Maybe something tragic happened in your life, and you felt like somehow you could have prevented it from happening. This can produce feelings of guilt that make you want to withdraw from others and protect your heart from further hurt. This reaction is normal but can be detrimental to you in the long run. Condemning yourself isn't healthy. Through Christ we have the ability to be forgiven for our sins and to move on.

In addition to feeling guilty, sadly I have found that many of us condemn ourselves. This condemnation brings feelings of shame. When we feel ashamed, many times we withdraw and close ourselves off from God and others. We even run away from those who love us the most and want to help us. We may feel as if we are powerless to remedy the situation we are in, and because of that, we turn to our drug of choice for comfort or numbing. The fat girl runs away from God and runs to food; the fit girl runs to Him for forgiveness, acceptance, and mercy.

The Bible says, "Therefore, there is now no condemnation for those who are in Christ Jesus, because through Christ Jesus the law of the Spirit of life set me free from the law of sin and death" (Romans 8:1-2). Sin brings death to us. This is a spiritual law. There are consequences for sin. But there is also good news! Jesus provided an escape from our guilt when He died for our sins. He set us free from the law of sin and death.

This may sound simplistic because it is something that we have heard all of our lives if we have been raised in church. But think about this. If it is so simple, then why do we still condemn ourselves? Why do we still run from God and His forgiveness rather than embrace Him? Why do we run to things like food for comfort rather than to God?

The important thing to remember when you are on the journey to becoming a fit girl is to recognize what makes you react in an overly emotional way and find ways to cope with those particular emotions. Take a minute right now and think about how you feel when you want to overindulge in food. What situations bring on those emotions for you? It doesn't have to be guilt or sadness; it can also be an emotion triggered by a pleasant memory. Whether it's attending a family reunion or party or passing by a favorite restaurant, only you can determine what those situations are. What makes you fall prey to the temptation of emotional eating?

In this chapter, I'll give you some tips to help you overcome this unhealthy eating pattern and modify your behavior to react differently.

Associating Food with Memories

Let me tell you a story about my mother. She spent a majority of her childhood being raised by my great-grandmother who had a unique name, Tiny Star Royston. Tiny lived on a farm in Royston, Georgia, with my Uncle Paul. I vaguely remember staying with them as a child. Tiny was getting older by then and died when I was only ten.

What I remember most about this time is the look of the farm. It boasted a white house with a wraparound front porch, complete with a swing and a few rocking chairs. The white paint on the house was chipped in places and weathered. The chicken coop, a long wooden building with a rusty, metal roof, housed noisy chickens.

The farm was located in a very rural area of Georgia. When we would go for a visit, we would drive down a long, dusty driveway before we actually got to the house. The beginning of the driveway was lined with tall cornstalks and looked like a fortress. As we drove farther on, huge gardens were planted on both sides of the driveway. It looked like the perfect setting for a movie.

My mother told me stories about how she and my great-grandmother spent the summers canning an endless variety of vegetables and fruits. She told me that Tiny always had a cake or a pie baked just in case company came to visit. The two of them sat on the rocking chairs on the front porch and entertained any guests who happened to stop by.

Though my mother was sad during this time because her parents divorced and she was left to be raised by her grandparents, Tiny gave her a sense of security and love. My mother held on dearly to the happy memories she shared with her grandmother. The thing was, many of those happy memories revolved around food. To this day, on holidays my mother loves to invite the whole family over to her house for a feast. She literally cooks for days preparing for Christmas, Thanksgiving, and Easter dinners. It's not enough to have turkey, dressing, and a few vegetables or side dishes. She sets out about ten items and usually about five desserts at each meal.

My mom is an excellent cook, and we always look forward to eating her tried-and-true recipes and getting a chance to taste new ones that she has discovered. To her, it isn't a holiday unless she is cooking.

Now, having a passion for cooking is not a bad thing. But it is a problem for my mother because she cooks with this fervor only around the holidays. To her, these special occasions are associated more with food than with the chance to spend time with loved ones. Like me, my mother has struggled with her weight all of her life. And it's obvious that food represents a celebration and conjures up some deep-seated emotions from her childhood.

How to Tell the Difference Between Hunger and Emotional Eating

There are several differences between emotional hunger and physical hunger, according to the University of Texas Counseling and Mental Health Center website.

1. Emotional hunger comes on suddenly; physical hunger occurs gradually.

2. When you are eating to fill a void that isn't related to an empty stomach, you crave a specific food, such as pizza or ice cream, and only that food will meet your need. When you eat because you are actually hungry, you're open to options.

3. Emotional hunger feels like it needs to be satisfied instantly with the food you crave; physical hunger can wait.

4. Even when you are full, if you're eating to satisfy an emotional need, you're more likely to keep eating. When you're eating because you're hungry, you're more likely to stop when you're full.

5. Emotional eating can leave behind feelings of guilt; eating when you are physically hungry does not.

If we think about it, most of us connect food to a happy celebration or holiday. What is the first word that comes to your mind when you think about cake? Is it "birthday"? I'll bet you anything it is! Gathering with friends and family around a cake, illuminated with glowing candles, and making a birthday wish is one of the happiest images I can think of. Birthdays are celebrations, and so when you eat cake, you have to be happy, right? Not necessarily, but that is what we have taught ourselves to believe.

The Problem with Holidays

When we are sad, it makes perfect sense that we turn to food to lift our spirits. If food reminds us of fun and memorable times (birthdays, Christmases, and Thanksgivings), the fat girl will believe that eating those foods will make her happier. Of course that's ridiculous, but those are the tapes we have created in our minds. And those tapes need to be reprogrammed.

Think about holidays. It seems at least once a month there is some kind of marked day that gives us permission to eat foods we know are not good for us. Not only that, but it seems that food is one of the highlights of the special occasion. Valentine's Day is about chocolate. Easter is about rabbit- or egg-shaped candy. The Fourth of July is about barbeques. Halloween is about candy. Thanksgiving is about, well, all kinds of food and gluttony. And Christmas is pretty much the same thing.

How can we not have a weight problem with all the celebrating we do? And how does a fit girl survive this madness?

Here is a picture of what our family holidays looked like when my fat girl was in control. We arrived at Mom's house a little before lunch. Before we sat down to eat, we snuck into the kitchen and tasted all of the delicious foods she prepared. Then we ate a hearty lunch followed by a generous helping (or two) of dessert. After a few hours of watching football or whatever else was on TV, we dug into another serving of food and then more dessert. Then we stretched out on the couch, rubbed our bellies, and complained of indigestion, bloating, and whatever else was ailing us because we ate too much.

How the Fit Girl Survives

The fit girl finds memorable traditions to use during the holidays that don't involve food. Here is an example. On Thanksgiving, our family's new tradition is to share, one by one, why we are thankful for each family member who is sitting around the table. We have also made it a habit to play games or puzzles after our meal. Then the children go outside and play, and the adults sit around and laugh and talk.

In a way, all these things signal that the time to eat is over. After our meal, there is something to look forward to besides food and more food. We look forward to spending time with each other. The more we focus on the people we are with and the love we have for them, the more we create happy emotions that have nothing to do with food.

Putting the fit girl in control also involves making healthier choices at holidays or celebrations. Where is it written in the rule books that we have to eat cake on our birthday or hot dogs on the Fourth of July? These are traditions we have lived with our whole lives, and, therefore, they have become what we do. There are always healthier alternatives we can choose. We can have turkey burgers instead of burgers made with beef. We can substitute small cupcakes for a huge birthday cake that we might be more tempted to eat too much of. We can use less butter and fat in the dishes we prepare.

People who live in the South are notorious for deep frying everything—even vegetables. Trust me. I know because I used to be one of them! It's normal for us to eat fried squash, okra, and even tomatoes. We also tend to use a lot of butter, shortening, and even bacon grease in many of our dishes. My mother used to keep a jar next to the stove, and every time she made bacon, she would pour the grease into the jar. She used it to make all kinds of things. She even put it in green beans!

It's no wonder holidays don't seem quite right to me without dishes that are laden with butter, cheese, and other things that aren't healthy for me. The fat girl would give herself a break over the holidays and pig out on these foods based on an emotional reaction to tradition. The fit girl, however, is not swayed by these emotions because she has the knowledge that keeping her body healthy is a choice she has to make every day.

This doesn't mean that she can never enjoy a treat. This just means that she keeps herself in check and modifies her choices when she can. I don't deprive myself of tasting something when I really want to; I just don't eat an excessive amount of it. If I see cake at a party, I might have a sliver instead of a huge slice. If someone offers me chocolate on Valentine's Day, I might have one piece instead of half the box.

One more thing. When I am asked to bring a dish to a holiday party, I make sure that what I bring is healthy. Here are some ideas I've incorporated into our family's celebrations.

- Birthday. Small cupcakes or angel food cake with strawberries instead of cake.
- Easter. Roast chicken or Cornish game hen instead of ham,

deviled eggs made with mustard and light mayonnaise instead of regular mayonnaise, and steamed green beans instead of beans with bacon grease.

- Fourth of July. Turkey burgers with mustard on whole wheat buns and spinach salad instead of ground beef burgers with white buns and potato salad.

- Thanksgiving. Steamed broccoli instead of broccoli with cheese sauce, steamed squash instead of fried squash, brown rice pilaf instead of stuffing or dressing, steamed carrots instead of glazed carrots, steamed green beans instead of green bean casserole, and fresh fruit with whipped topping rather than pumpkin pie.

- Christmas. Whole, baked sweet potatoes instead of candied yams, fresh fruit instead of fruit cake, peppermint tea rather than candy canes, wheat pasta salad instead of macaroni and cheese, turkey or grilled chicken instead of ham, and grilled asparagus instead of fried okra.

I also try to think about ways to give gifts that aren't food. For example, rather than give candy to my husband or children for Halloween, Valentine's Day, or Easter, I give them little gifts, toys, or a book.

These are just a few things the fit girl might do to stop associating the holidays with emotions and food. You might have a couple more ideas in mind.

The main thing to remember is that just because you have always done something one way, it doesn't mean you have to continue to do it that way. Have you heard the saying, "If you always do what you've always done, you will always get what you've always got"? This is true with many things in life. If you do the same things over and over, you will produce the same results.

The fit girl knows that her emotional reactions to food have to change to be fit. She has to go against what she has always done to get a good, healthy result.

Help! This Seems Too Hard!

I know for some of you, I may have attacked something sacred in your life. You may be reading this chapter and thinking, *Oh my goodness, Amy. Really? I have to rethink attaching emotions to food and even holidays? But Christmas is not Christmas without Aunt Ruth's sweet potato pie. I don't know if I can do it!*

Let me tell you something. That kind of reaction is what can keep you from your destiny. If you are hesitant to change, you may be substituting a longer life and a healthy fulfilling future for a tradition or emotional attachment to food. Is food more important than your health? I don't think so.

Here are some tips to combat emotional eating:

- Manage your moods! Making note of the mood you are in when you run to the fridge is a good way to determine what mood you are in when you are tempted to overeat.

- Monitor your emotions daily. Checking your emotional levels daily can help you trace the reasons why you indulge in emotional eating and can help you solve these emotions before beginning any meal. This can also help you fight the urge to overeat when you get emotionally upset.

- Be a busy bee. Try to develop new interests and hobbies that will take your mind off food. By keeping yourself busy, you can avoid eating and snacking out of boredom.

- Work out a meal plan you know you will stick with. Having a solid plan in mind will prevent you from grabbing food on impulse.

- Work it out. Physical activity can help your body burn unwanted calories and lower your stress levels. Exercise also releases positive endorphins, and those help you fight depression.

- Develop closer friendships and emotional bonds. Having a friend or group of friends who can give you moral support will help you combat negative emotions. Just talking with a girlfriend can release stress and help you deal with things better.

- Draw closer to God. A closer relationship with God fills a place inside that nothing else can. Laying down your burdens through prayer is a great way to deal with stress.

- Drink your water! Drink at least eight glasses of water daily to keep your body refreshed and well hydrated so you won't easily get irritated or upset.

- Choose your treats wisely. Comfort foods such as junk foods should be replaced with healthier alternatives.

- Learn to forgive yourself. When you blow your diet, forgive yourself. Feeling guilty and depressed will only make matters worse. Instead of dwelling on your failures, try to be positive by telling yourself you can do better tomorrow.

You may also be saying to yourself, *The fit girl is asking too much of me. This is too hard of a sacrifice!* Or you may think, *But I'm not strong enough to make all of those changes in my life.*

Stop right there. I believe that you are a strong, courageous person. I believe that you can do whatever it takes to get the things out of life that you truly need and want. If you are a mother, think about your children for a minute. Every mom wants what is best for her children. I'm sure you will sacrifice and do whatever it takes to meet your kids' needs. If you are a friend, think about this. If a friend really needs you, you will move heaven and earth to be there for them. If you're married, think about your spouse. Wouldn't you drop whatever you are doing if he has an emergency and needs you? Yes. Yes. Yes!

As women, most of us take care of everyone else all of the time, and guess who ends up being the person at the bottom of the totem pole? That's right. You! You don't give yourself enough credit; just like you probably don't take enough time to take care of yourself.

You are powerful in ways that you can't even imagine. You are an amazing creature. You work hard and love soft. You survive and thrive. You fight and nurture. And you know what else? You are strong enough to fight the fat-girl fight and win! That's right!

When you start thinking you can't win this war because your emotional reactions to food are too strong, you are not letting God be in control of all areas of your life. Ephesians 4:17-24 says:

> So I tell you this, and insist on it in the Lord, that you must no longer live as the Gentiles do, in the futility of their thinking. They are darkened in their understanding and separated from the life of God because of the ignorance that is in them due to the hardening of their hearts. Having lost all sensitivity, they have given themselves over to sensuality so as to indulge in every kind of impurity, with a continual lust for more.
>
> You, however, did not come to know Christ that way. Surely you heard of him and were taught in him in accordance with the truth that is in Jesus. You were taught, with regard to your former way of life, to put off your old self, which is being corrupted by its deceitful desires; to be made new in the attitude of your minds; and to put on the new self, created to be like God in true righteousness and holiness.

The Power of God Is in You to Do All Things

This passage of Scripture describes how we should live our lives as Christians. We should be strong and powerful knowing that through Christ we have the power to overcome the desires of our flesh. We know that we "can do all things through Christ who strengthens" us as it says in Philippians 4:13 (one of my favorite verses). The power to change is within you. You have the power through Christ to make the changes and see results. You have the power to make choices that make your life better or worse. God has given us that power, even at the risk of losing us.

I remember the first time I felt like I understood God's relationship with humankind and the principles of redemption. I was in a Bible class, and the professor was teaching on the story of Adam and Eve. He said when God created Adam, God didn't want him to be like anything else He created. So He gave Adam free will. He gave him the power to choose between right and wrong.

Adam was free to do anything he wanted in the Garden of Eden. He had a paradise to live in, all the food he could eat, and a beautiful wife. God told him there was only one rule—he couldn't eat from the tree of knowledge of good and evil. (God started off small; He created only one way the first human beings could possibly sin, and it involved food as a temptation!) I imagine God standing back and watching Adam and Eve with bated breath. *Choosing to obey Me above the temptation of sin is a very difficult choice.* And, yet, He trusted His children to do the right thing.

We all know the story. Eve ate from the tree after being deceived by the serpent, and Adam followed suit. Then God called them out on what they had done. God knew that they had done something wrong and saw that they were ashamed. Shame did not exist before this moment, but sin brought it into the world. Instead of humbling himself, Adam blamed God and said something like, "If it wasn't for that darn woman you gave me…"

I'm sure God was disappointed, but the next part of the story is where you realize how precious we are to Him. He had already created a contingency plan to redeem humankind. See, when Adam and Eve sinned, they basically gave the lease of the whole earth over to Satan. But all along, God had plans to redeem the world. He planned to come to earth as a man, live a perfect life, and die on a cross. The shedding of His blood was the price needed to "buy back" the earth that Adam sold through sin. God was willing to die to make up for our screwups.

This should bring you hope if you are struggling in the area of emotional eating. Through Christ we can start over today to make good choices. We don't have to sell ourselves or our future short through the lust of the flesh when it comes to food. If you accept God's gift of redemption through Christ, then the power of God lives in you!

Adam failed in his own strength to stand against his desires so God gave His strength to Adam. The Bible talks about this in Romans 8:5-11. "Those who live according to the sinful nature have their minds set on what that nature desires; but those who live in accordance with the Spirit have their minds set on what the Spirit desires. The mind of sinful man is death, but the mind controlled by the Spirit is life and peace; the sinful mind is hostile to God. It does not submit to God's law, nor can it do so. Those controlled by the sinful nature cannot please God. You, however, are controlled not by the sinful nature but by the Spirit, if the Spirit of God lives in you. And if anyone does not have the Spirit of Christ, he does not belong to Christ. But if Christ is in you, your body is dead because of sin, yet your spirit is alive because of righteousness. And if the Spirit of him who raised Jesus from the dead is living in you, he who raised Christ from the dead will also give life to your mortal bodies through his Spirit, who lives in you."

We used to sing a song in church based on Romans 8:9. It went something like this:

> If the same spirit that raised Christ from the dead
>   dwells in you,
> He dwells in you,
> He will quicken your mortal body,
> If that Spirit dwells in you.

At the time, I didn't really understand how all that applied to me personally. Now I realize that this song and this passage tell me that the power of Christ lives inside of me. I am strong, not because of my strength but because the power of the Creator of the universe lives in my spirit. How can an emotional attachment to food be stronger than the One who created food? That's just silly!

❦ TRANSFORMATION TIPS ❦

Rise up and realize how strong and powerful you are through Christ. Realize food cannot control your emotions unless you allow it to do so. Allow the power of Christ to work in your life in this area. Trust Him to give you the power you need to make the changes necessary to deal with your emotions instead of running to food to cope.

1. What are some emotions you connect to food? What are three ways you can prevent those emotions from controlling you?

2. On what holidays do you feel especially vulnerable? Write down three ways to substitute unhealthy traditions for healthier ones, so you don't associate a holiday function with food.

3. Examine your relationship with God and food. Is God in control, or is food in control?

4. When do you feel weak and need God's power to help? Read Philippians 4:19. How does this verse encourage you?

❦ Your Prayer ❦

Lord, thank You for living in me and giving me the strength I need to overcome the challenges that come my way. I pray for power and control over food. I pray that You would remind me that I do not have to attach emotion to food or make it the center of attention on special occasions. I pray that You help me see food for what it is—something to nourish my body, which is a temple created for Your glory. Thank You for Your strength and might. Thank You that I am able to do all things because of—and only because of—You. In Jesus' name I pray. Amen.

Your Thoughts

Food Is Not a Stress Buster

There are very few certainties that touch us all in this mortal experience, but one of the absolutes is that we will experience hardship and stress at some point.

—Dr. James C. Dobson

When I was about 11 years old, I had a ritual that I often did. I would look under the cushions of the sofa or in my mother's old purses for loose change. When I found a sufficient amount, I walked to the neighborhood convenience store. When I got there, I surveyed the candy aisle with excitement and looked for the prized treat that I was going to take home with me. Usually I purchased a king-sized bag of M&Ms or a chocolate bar. After that I returned home, found a blanket, sat on the sofa, and watched—here is where I age myself—*Bewitched, My Three Sons,* and *Three's Company.*

I ate the candy very slowly, savoring every bite and trying really hard to make it last through all three shows. This was my release from the turmoil in my family. Eating treats while watching TV washed away all the cares of the day. It was complete relaxation and, like a drug, it gave me such a great feeling that I wanted to do it over and over again. And I did—for years.

What's Your Unwinding Pleasure?

To this day when I watch one of my favorite television shows, especially after a long, hard day, I find myself wanting to have some kind of sweet snack to eat. I always think to myself, *This show is great, but it would be so much better with a dessert.* I know that watching a favorite television show is one of the triggers that compels me to crave sweets. It's a connection I have developed since I was a girl, and it's something I have had to overcome.

Though the fat girl conditions herself to use food as a means of unwinding, the fit girl recognizes that food is not a stress buster and uses other methods to unwind. The fat girl gives in and eats, thinking that the food is going to make her feel better, calmer, and less stressed. The fit girl is aware of stressful situations that will cause her to be tempted and develops strategies to help her overcome the temptation.

Relaxing with food is definitely a habit that can be difficult to break. In many ways, it's tougher to control than a drug addiction. One reason is obvious—we have to eat to live. Drug addicts and alcoholics can live without their drug for the rest of their lives. Food addicts don't have that same luxury. They need to eat.

Fit-Girl Options

As a former fat girl, I know how tough it is to not use food to relax—tough but not impossible. I think the most important thing to learn is how to deal with stress in ways that have nothing to do with eating. We can find things to do that can help us relax. Listen, as long as we're alive, stress isn't going to disappear. In today's fast-paced world, we are constantly juggling family, friends, faith, career, health, and, of course, ourselves. It's a tough act to do successfully. But as a fit girl, it's easier to do when you have strategies in place to deal with the urge to overeat, eat when you're not hungry, or use food as a coping mechanism.

Techniques to Reduce Stress

1. Practice letting go of the things that bother you. Imagine that those things that keep nagging at you are balloons you are letting go of. They float up into the sky to never be seen again. This helps when people say things to you that bother you or if a problem comes up that is difficult. Don't dwell on those things; just let them go.

2. Breathe slowly and deeply. Have you ever noticed how when you get stressed, you involuntarily sigh? This is because your body is trying to help you to release tension. Before reacting to the next stressful situation, take three deep breaths and release them slowly.

3. Practice speaking slower than usual. You'll find that when you do this, you think more clearly and react more reasonably to stressful situations. When you speak slowly, you force the rest of your reactions to slow down as well. When you slow down your speech, you'll also appear less anxious and more in control of any situation.

4. Jump-start a time management plan. Choose one thing you have been putting off (returning a phone call, scheduling a doctor's appointment, or something else), and do it immediately. Just taking care of one nagging responsibility can be energizing and improve your attitude.

5. Get some fresh air! It is true that fresh air can clear your mind and energize you. Even five minutes outside can be refreshing. So take five!

6. Drink plenty of water and eat small, nutritious snacks. Hunger and dehydration, even before you're aware of them, can exacerbate feelings of anxiety.

7. Sit up straight! There is a reason why our parents told us this. Hold your head and shoulders upright and avoid stooping or slumping. Bad posture can lead to muscle tension, pain, and increased stress.

8. Plan to treat yourself or get a reward at the end of your stressful day, even if only a relaxing bath or half an hour with a good book. Put aside work and housekeeping a few hours before bedtime and allow yourself to fully relax. Don't spend this time planning tomorrow's schedule or doing chores you didn't get around to doing during the day. Remember that you need time to recharge and energize yourself. You will be better prepared to handle things when you have time for yourself.

I'll talk a lot about these strategies throughout this chapter, but here are some things to think about. Everyone has a different way of relaxing or unwinding that can be just as powerful as a candy bar, potato chips, or chocolate. Some women love taking bubble baths. Some get a massage. Some read books. Some go for a walk. Some make a cup of tea or coffee and sit outdoors. There are many ways to relax that don't involve mindless munching.

Matthew 5:29 tells us, "If your right eye causes you to sin, gouge it out and throw it away. It is better for you to lose one part of your body than for your whole body to be thrown into hell." This verse is figuratively saying that if a part of our body is causing us to sin, we should get rid of it. Obviously, this is not a literal suggestion. We can't chop off our hand or foot. That would be foolish, not to mention painful. We can, however, anticipate when we are going to be in situations that will tempt us to sin and avoid those situations, or if we can't avoid them, we can learn how to deal with them in a healthy way.

I didn't think giving up watching a TV show at night before bed was going to work for me, so I had to figure out a way to avoid being tempted to eat something unhealthy during that time. I found what works for me. On the nights I watch my show of choice, I purposely exercise later in the afternoon or in the early evening. Doing some form of cardio, like running, helps to release the stress of the day. Rigorous exercise, especially cardio, also suppresses my appetite. The endorphins that are released during this activity calm me down and keep me from needing food to relax.

Stress-Buster Exercises

Use these exercises at home or work when you are confronted with a stressful situation.

1. Squeeze it out! Get a stress ball—a thick foam ball that's made to be squeezed in your hand. Squeezing one during times of tension will help you direct your negative feelings toward the ball instead of a bag of candy.

2. Resist the urge to go to the drive-thru! Instead, exercise with resistance bands. Use resistance bands at home or at your desk to tone your arms and relieve stress at the same time.

3. Walk it out! Get up and take a power walk around your house or run the stairs in your office building to get those positive endorphins going.

4. Stand up and stretch! Take a few minutes every day to stretch your arms over your head. This will release tension in your shoulders, back, and neck.

5. Hit something! Taking a boxing class is a good way to release stress and aggression. If something is bothering me, I imagine hitting that problem and knocking it out. You can also purchase and hang up a punching bag in your home or office to use anytime you are feeling particularly tense.

If I'm physically hungry, I choose healthy snacks like frozen grapes or air-popped popcorn with a little sugar-free chocolate syrup drizzled on it. Sometimes I freeze small cups of yogurt and eat it like ice cream. (Greek yogurt is a great option because it has more protein and less sugar than other kinds.) Sometimes I add a little cocoa, xylitol (a natural sweetener), natural peanut butter, or almond butter to it before I freeze it. As long as it fits into my calorie budget, I'm good to go!

7 Stress-Busting Foods

- Oatmeal: Carbohydrates make the brain produce more serotonin, the same relaxing brain chemical released when you eat dark chocolate. Oatmeal is also full of fiber and gives you that full feeling.

- Oranges: The magic nutrient here is vitamin C. In a study in *Psychopharmacology*, German researchers subjected 120 people to a public-speaking task plus a series of math problems. Those who took 3000 milligrams of vitamin C reported that they felt less stressed, and their blood pressure and levels of cortisol (a stress hormone) returned to normal faster.

- Salmon: Stress hormones have an archenemy—omega-3 fatty acids. A 2003 study from *Diabetes & Metabolism* found that a diet rich in omega-3 fatty acids kept cortisol and adrenaline from going into overload. Omega-3 fatty acids also protect against heart disease, according to a 2002 study in the *Journal of the American Medical Association*.

- Spinach: Magnesium is prevalent in spinach and is the mineral that can help lower your stress levels, keeping your body in a state of relative ease. Not getting enough magnesium may trigger migraine headaches and make you feel fatigued. Just one cup of spinach provides 40 percent of your daily value. Try substituting it for lettuce on sandwiches and salads too.

- Almonds, Pistachios, and Walnuts: When it all breaks loose, reach for a handful of almonds. They're bursting with vitamin E, an antioxidant that bolsters the immune system. Almonds also contain B vitamins, which may help your body hold up during unpleasant events. About a quarter cup every day is all you need. Throw them on salads or in yogurt too. Another easy way to get a fix is to switch from traditional peanut butter to almond butter on high-tension days. Pistachios and walnuts are also great nuts to choose from as well.

- Avocados: The next time stress has you hankering for a treat, try some homemade guacamole. This delicious treat contains monounsaturated fat and potassium, which can lower blood pressure. One of the best ways to reduce high blood pressure, according to the National Heart, Lung, and Blood Institute, is to get enough potassium. Just half an avocado offers 487 milligrams; more than you'll get from a medium-sized banana.

- Skim Milk: Science backs up the old warm-milk remedy for insomnia and restlessness. It turns out that calcium can reduce muscle spasms and soothe tension. A glass of milk (preferably skim or 1 percent) may also reduce stressful PMS symptoms, such as mood swings, anxiety, and irritability. According to a 2005 study from the *Archives of Internal Medicine*, women who drank four or more servings of low-fat or skim milk per day had a 46 percent lower risk of preperiod misery than women who had no more than one serving per week.

Feeling Overwhelmed?

During my journey to become a fit girl, I have found that not only did I use food to unwind, but I also used it to cope with stress. If I'm feeling overwhelmed about having a lot of things to do, my immediate reaction is to eat. Feeling powerless over a hectic schedule and a lengthy to-do list makes me restless. This is when I have the tendency to turn to food for some kind of stimulation.

Learning how to better manage my time and organize the details of my life helps me cope with this issue. I use a monthly calendar to write down everything I need to do and remember. I jot down even the smallest things, like calling a friend, writing a thank-you note, or taking the trash to the curb. Doing this—rather than leaving those tasks to just float around inside my head—makes me feel less overwhelmed by all the things I have to do. Also, when I write them down, I don't worry about forgetting something. I can categorize the items from the most important to the least important. I enjoy checking each one off after I have done them. It makes me feel as though I've accomplished something.

I especially like organizing my lists at night when I need to wind down from the day. It helps me get a good night's sleep because those thoughts are now out of my mind and on my list. I can close the door on them, knowing they will be taken care of tomorrow (or the next day).

I also keep a calendar on my cell phone, so I can input appointments as they come up. This is great because I can program an alarm to remind me of upcoming meetings, deadlines, or appointments. I never worry about forgetting to show up somewhere or get something done. Being more organized and schedule-oriented helps me feel more in control of my life. It also makes me feel less tempted to get stimulation from food.

Maybe you are like me and get anxious when you see disorder and chaos in your life. I think most women do. I want to challenge you to get better organized. Go to your local library or bookstore and check out books on this subject. There are many great ones out there that will help you better organize your time, your money, your schedule, your family, and even your home.

Speaking of home, I heard someone once say that if your closet is unorganized and it's the first place you go to in the morning, the state of that space will set the tone for your whole day. So, what does your closet look like? Are your clothes hung up nice and neat? Or are they strewn all over the floor, so you can't tell what's clean or dirty? When I have my closets and even my kitchen and bathroom cabinets organized, I feel more relaxed and calmer. Take some time to put your house in order. I guarantee it will help relieve some of the stress or restlessness you may be feeling.

Make Peace at Home

I have always been a Type A personality. I want to go 90 miles an hour until I literally drop to the floor from exhaustion. My husband is the opposite. He paces himself and slowly and methodically does his work. He always knows to rest and take a break when he's tired. My mother calls us the racehorse and the Clydesdale. The problem with Clydesdales is they don't move fast enough for the racehorses.

This imbalance can occasionally cause stress in my life. Don't get me wrong. I love Phillip and know he is my perfect match. I believe God puts opposites together to complement each other. But let's be honest. Sometimes those opposite traits can get on each other's nerves. When I am frustrated because Phillip doesn't move fast enough for me, or if there is tension between us for any other reason, I can be tempted to run to the pantry or fridge to unwind.

In this situation I have learned to be a better communicator of my needs and wants. I believe many of us expect our loved ones to read our minds and know what we want or need them to do. I'm guilty as charged. Sometimes I think that after being married for 20 years, Phillip should always anticipate what I need and do it. But that's just ridiculous!

It took a while for me to understand that though Phillip wants to help and provide for me, he has to either see my request in writing (like a cute note) or hear me ask him in a respectful, kind, and warm way. Barking orders at him or giving him the silent treatment because he didn't do what I wanted is counterproductive. And that causes more stress.

I am learning what it takes to make a peaceful home. Keeping peace in my marriage by using effective communication is a key to preventing a desire to eat to unwind. Less stress in our home equals less overeating. I know this is not always easy, but trust me, it is doable.

From TV to the Real World

When I came home from The Biggest Loser Ranch, I had a tough time figuring out how to do everything at home. You have to remember that on the ranch, working out and eating healthy is your full-time job. I had lived in a "weight-loss wonderland" for two and a half months, and coming home to the real world was quite a shock. At the ranch, you don't have the distractions of children, work, bills, telephones, televisions, or anything else. In fact, you don't even know what is going on in the world because there are no radios, magazines, or newspapers.

When I came home, I was instantly bombarded with all of these things and felt extremely overwhelmed. On top of that, I now had people from all over the country emailing me weight-loss questions. I wanted to help them, so I would take time out to try to answer each one. The depressed real estate market was another challenge I faced. I worked in the industry, but because of the economy, we had to figure out how to support our family and pay our bills another way.

Many times I was so wound up, I felt like my nerve endings were going to pop out of my body. For a fat girl who had always turned to food to unwind, I was faced with the ultimate battle. I had to figure out new ways to cope with my stress because I had traveled too far to get sidetracked. I quickly discovered that running on the treadmill while listening to my iPod was a great way to release some of the tension. It didn't fix everything, but it was a good start.

I didn't love running at first. I had to convince myself that I loved to run so that it would be a positive experience and something I craved rather than dreaded. I did this by telling myself things like, *Yeah! I get to exercise today. Being on this treadmill is my idea. No one else is making me do this. I am able to.* I looked at working out as a privilege; something I was *able* to do rather than something that *had* to be done.

Many times, simply changing your outlook can make whatever is difficult easier. You can actually talk yourself into liking something that you once hated. You can change your belief system when it comes to things that are healthy for you.

During this time of transition, I also realized that eating properly and regularly is crucial. If I went too long without eating, I would find myself having overwhelming cravings. I kept a food journal in which I wrote down what I ate and when.

Here are two of the most important tips, which I still use today to keep my eating under control, lessen my cravings, and keep my triggers at bay: 1) Combine proteins, carbohydrates, and a healthy fat with every meal; 2) eat every three to four hours like clockwork. Eating this way regulates your blood sugar levels and gives you sustained energy throughout the day. Keeping blood sugar levels steady is important to combat nasty cravings that make it almost impossible not to overeat during times of stress. These two tips are major fit-girl weapons in my arsenal against eating to unwind.

We All Need Support

Another tip that helped me during that time was to develop a good support system. Let me start by saying that I am not the kind of person who likes to ask people for help. I am a do-it-yourself kind of girl. I will overwork myself, get frustrated, and stressed out because I never ask for help.

I was constantly stressed as a fat girl because I never wanted to inconvenience anyone, and so I never let anyone know what I needed. My husband is more of a delegator. He is constantly seeing what he can get someone else to do, so he can be more productive. It was hard for me, but while adjusting to regular life, I was forced to learn how to delegate.

When Phillip and I were chosen to be on *The Biggest Loser,* I discovered that so many people were willing to help us. We had a wonderful friend and fellow realtor named Lisa who helped us with our real estate listings. We will be eternally grateful to her for all of her hard work. We had many people volunteer to help us with our children too. My sister-in-law and sisters were godsends because they watched our boys. Our grandparents became involved as well. We actually inherited many "grandparents" who took our kids to the movies and out to eat. Our boys became closer to our extended family during this journey because they spent so much more time with them.

Our trainers, like DJ Jordan, who became like a member of the family, gave us so much support. We had neighbors who helped us with things around the house, like watering our plants and cutting the grass. It was amazing to see so many people rally around to help us during this time. They alleviated so much stress and enabled me to continue my journey toward health and success. I will never be able to repay these people for all they did for us. I will be forever indebted to them for their kindness.

I know that my situation was a little extreme because I was in a weight-loss competition on a reality show. You may be thinking that there is no way you could get the same kind of support system. I disagree. I believe that you have more supportive people in your life than you realize. You have family and friends who care about your well-being. They want you to be healthy and see you transform from the fat girl into the fit girl.

Pray and ask God to show you who those people are. Reach outside of your comfort zone and ask people for help. If you are like me, it might be a difficult thing to do. That's okay! It's part of the growing process. If you reach out, I'm sure you will be pleasantly surprised at the response you receive.

Don't Forget About You

Here's another big pointer to alleviating stress. I found that as a fat girl, I always did everything for everyone else and put myself dead last. By doing this, I was stuck in a vicious cycle. I tended to everyone else's needs, and by the time the day was over, I crashed on the sofa to eat and watch TV. Sound familiar? Most women have a tough time taking care of themselves. We want to be the best wife, mother, sister, and friend. We want to volunteer and work full-time. We want to raise perfect children. We want to keep a perfect house. We want to have order in all corners of our house. We want to do for everyone, and when it comes time for ourselves, we don't have any energy left.

The fat girl always puts herself last. The fit girl takes care of herself so that she has energy to help care for her loved ones. My children and husband had always relied on me to do things for them that they really should have been doing themselves. It wasn't their fault for relying on me so much. I had actually trained them with my actions to behave that way. I remember that before meals I would cut up their meat into tiny pieces, and then after meals, I would go from one to another around the table with a wet paper towel to make sure their hands were clean. How crazy is that? Uh-oh, maybe you do the same thing!

The fit girl realized that doing all of this kept them from growing up and added more (and unnecessary) stress to her life. When I transformed into a fit girl, my children learned how to take on more responsibility. No longer was Mom picking up after them all the time. They learned to clean their own rooms, take out the trash, do the dishes, and vacuum. I always joke about when they get married, their wives will love me because I taught them how to do housework. Phillip was a great asset. He learned how to wash, fold, and iron his own clothes. We work together on the household chores now. Our home environment has changed in this process. It is a healthy and less stressful place to live.

One way to help you take care of yourself is to incorporate a particular word into your vocabulary—"boundaries." We all need to establish boundaries with friends and family and learn to say no when necessary. As a fat girl, I never wanted to tell anyone no because I wanted everyone to like me. I thought if I said no, something catastrophic would happen, and so I continued to say yes with a smile on my face. But as this was happening, I was going crazy inside.

How many times do we say yes when we really should be saying no? Some of the most successful people in this world know how to set limits and maintain boundaries. I was privileged to be a guest on an episode of the *Oprah Show* titled "Life Makeovers." When I met her, I was most impressed with how firm her boundaries are. Everyone loves Oprah, and yet she sets limits on everything. She could spend every waking hour taking pictures with people or answering letters, but she is very selective about who she lets into her circle and what causes she supports.

This taught me a valuable lesson. People do not value you when you are so easily accessible. They value you when you set limits. While

I thought saying yes made people like me more, it actually made them appreciate me less. I allowed myself to be taken advantage of by agreeing to do things, be somewhere, and meet with people when I didn't have the time or the energy.

Listen, fit girls, we don't have to do everything all the time. We have to choose what will ultimately bring value to our time, our priorities, our future, our sanity, and our well-being. We are treasures, and we need to treat ourselves as such. We need to learn to say no to the people and things that are not a priority in our lives. Saying yes all the time will keep us busy and stressed twenty-four hours a day. Who wants to live like that? The fit girl certainly doesn't!

❦ TRANSFORMATION TIPS ❦

Are you ready to keep stress away? Are you ready to sever your association with food and stress? Here are some reminders about what you've read so far to help keep you on track:

- Find alterative ways to relax that don't involve eating. Take a trip, go for a walk, or take a hot bath.
- Improve your organizational and time-management skills. Disorder is stressful; order is relaxing.
- Work on your communication skills. Instead of getting frustrated because your needs are not being met, learn to better express your needs to those who can help you with them.
- Develop a support system. When you can, delegate tasks to others.
- Take time for yourself.
- Learn how to say no. Set limits on people, tasks, and other things.

Regarding the six suggestions listed above, how can you use these tips to make your life less stressful?

Now think of three things you can do to relax that don't involve food. Write down your ideas, post the list on the refrigerator or pantry door, and let them remind you of healthy ways to relax.

What are some disorderly areas in your life? What are some things you can do to change those areas? Maybe your closet is cluttered, and you need to take a weekend to organize it. Maybe you need to buy a planner and write your schedule down. Whatever it is, commit to changing one thing this week.

What are some things with which you could use some help? Maybe you need to hire a housekeeper or a babysitter. Think of people who might be able to help you. Call one person this week and ask for help.

⋙ Your Prayer ⋘

*Father, thank You for calling me to live an abundant
and peaceful life—not a life of stress. Show me how
I can manage my stress better and even eliminate
unnecessary stress in particular areas. Give me
creative ideas and strategies to overcome the areas
in my life that cause me to feel overwhelmed. Help
me live with peace in my heart, so I can exude that
peace to those I love. In Jesus' name I pray. Amen.*

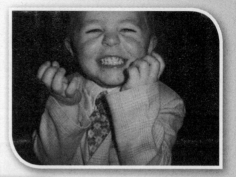

Rhett—before he was diagnosed with autism

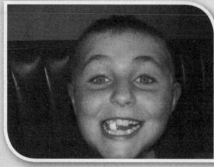

Rhett now

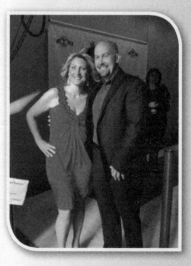

Phillip and me—walking the red carpet

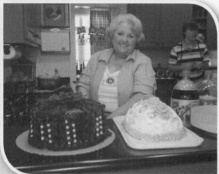

My sweet little mama. Look at all those desserts! No wonder I struggle with weight!

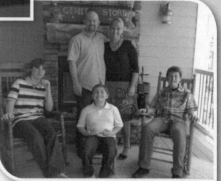

My little family

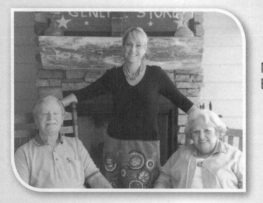

Mama, my stepfather Bill, and me

My sister Allyson, me, and other sister Donna

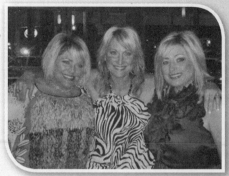

Phillip and me— at Phillip's first half marathon

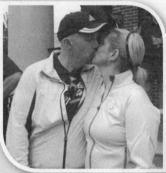

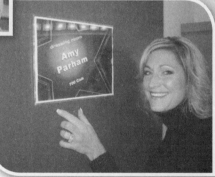

My dressing room at *The 700 Club* taping

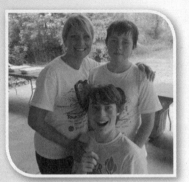

My older boys, Austin and Pearson, and me—at a bike race

Ally, my daddy, and me

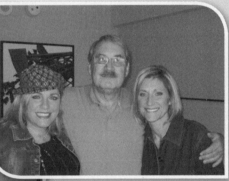

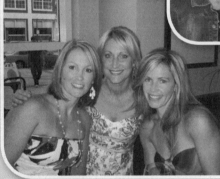

My skinny sister-in-law Joan, me, and our friend Toni

Fitness Is Your Friend

*I don't exercise. If God had wanted me to bend
over, he would have put diamonds on the floor.*

—JOAN RIVERS

Other than taking a co-ed weightlifting class in college (for reasons that entirely involved gawking at the male members of the class), I never darkened the door of a gym before I arrived at The Biggest Loser Ranch. I'll never forget that first day on the campus.

Walking into the gym was overwhelming. The room looked like a medieval dungeon full of torture devices. I had no clue how to operate any of the machines. I was particularly terrified of the treadmill because the fat girl in me was naturally clumsy and had a horrible sense of balance and rhythm. Although the first time I stepped on it, I feigned enthusiasm, after I walked for a few more minutes, I suddenly found myself genuinely beaming with pride.

Unfortunately, it didn't take long for my bubble to burst. "Amy, why are you holding onto that treadmill?" my trainer, Bob, asked. I looked at him, bewildered, and replied, "Aren't you supposed to?" My question was met with laughter from everyone around me. Apparently everyone except me knew you weren't supposed to hold onto the side bars. How was I supposed to know? I had never been a gym member. I hadn't ever really worked out before.

Not being able to hold on to the bars of the treadmill ripped away my last shred of what little confidence I had. There I was in a hot gym, completely out of my comfort zone, and now I actually had to balance on this treadmill? The thought frightened me. I wanted to run away. However, I knew I couldn't waste any energy being afraid. I had to save my energy for working out for hours a day. I was given the incredible opportunity to be on *The Biggest Loser,* and I certainly was not going to let my fear of exercise stand in the way of my success. I had to make the choice to conquer this mountain that stood between me and the fit girl.

Guess what happened? Before I knew it, I was walking on the treadmill for hours at a time. (Look, Mom, no hands!) Soon after that, I started running for a few minutes at a time. Gradually I built up the time to 30 minutes and then an hour. Soon I began to actually look forward to exercise. All of this happened within a matter of weeks. Through this process, I finally realized what the fit girl understands—exercise is a friend.

The Difference Exercise Makes

The fat girl has a million excuses (and some even seem pretty good) why you can't exercise. She knows that if you exercise regularly, you will feel strong, and the fat girl won't have the power anymore. Well, in this case, the fat girl is right!

Exercise is important for several reasons. It's good for you physically, mentally, and emotionally. You can use this block of time to focus on yourself. When I exercise, I deal with stress better and feel much more energetic. I can tell when I haven't taken time to exercise regularly. I get emotional and moody. Taking time to be active regulates my inner well-being by creating endorphins that help me feel calm.

When I was a newlywed, Phillip and I took a trip to New York to attend his sister's wedding. My soon to be brother-in-law's family was gracious enough to take us on a sightseeing tour of Manhattan for a day. I was so excited to see all that the city had to offer—in fact, it was a dream come true—but I had no idea how much exercise would be involved. We walked from place to place all day, only occasionally stopping to ride the subway.

At the time, I was in my early twenties, and although I was not overweight, I still struggled the entire day to keep up with the rest of the group. When I should have been enjoying the city that I had always dreamed of seeing, I was thinking, *When can we go home?* I was sore the next day and wondered how the people who lived there could possibly walk everywhere all the time.

Recently, Phillip and I went back to New York City. Though 20 years had passed and we'd gotten older, you wouldn't believe the difference! One morning we took a run from our hotel to Central Park and then continued running throughout the park. We spent the rest of the day walking all over the city sightseeing, and then we walked back to our hotel. I never struggled—not even for a minute—and had plenty of energy the whole day. What a difference being physically active made during our second trip to the Big Apple!

The biggest difference I have experienced since I started exercising regularly is the increase in energy. As a fat girl, I used to feel perpetually tired. I used to think that exercise burns energy, so if you don't exercise, you would have extra energy, right? Wrong. When you exercise regularly, you will notice your energy levels increasing!

10 Tips to Help You Stay on the Plan

1. Follow an effective exercise routine. Make sure that when you are working out, you are doing exercises that make a difference. The American Council on Exercise (ACE) recently surveyed 1000 ACE-certified personal trainers about the best techniques to get fit. Here are their top three suggestions:

   • Strength training. Even 20 minutes a day twice a week will help tone the entire body.

   • Interval training. "In its most basic form, interval

training might involve walking for two minutes, running for two, and alternating this pattern throughout the duration of a workout," says Cedric Bryant, PhD, FACSM, chief science officer for ACE. "It is an extremely time-efficient and productive way to exercise."

- Increased cardio/aerobic exercise. Bryant suggests accumulating 60 minutes or more a day of low- to moderate-intensity physical activity, such as walking, running, or dancing.

2. Set goals you can reach. We have all made goals like "I am going lose 20 pounds in a week" or "I am going to fit into a bikini by summer." These lofty types of goals are dangerous when it comes to exercise. Setting unrealistic exercise goals like "I am going to run a 5K in a month" when you have never even walked a mile, can be counterproductive over the long term. Make attainable short-term goals. As you master them, gradually set longer-term goals that require more effort. This plan will help you stick with your exercise plan over the long haul.

3. Take a friend with you. Having a friend to work out with provides an accountability factor and makes exercise more fun. For me if I didn't have friends or my trainer counting on me to show up, some mornings it would be far easier to roll over and go back to sleep. Pick a friend who is at the same fitness level as you are and will push you to reach your goals.

4. Consistency counts. When you start moving, your body doesn't stop! Exercising consistently is as important as what exercises you do. Even though you may not run miles each day, you will soon see results if you consistently do some kind of effective exercise routine each day.

5. Do activities you look forward to. If you love the outdoors, you might want to choose hiking, biking, or swimming. If you like to be around people, you might want to

try group fitness classes. If you do something that you love, you are more likely to continue doing it.

6. Watch your energy levels. Are you are morning person who loves to get up with the chickens? Then you may want to work out in the morning. Do you find that you can't get going in the morning but have a lot of energy as the day goes on? Then maybe you should schedule your workouts during the afternoon or evening. Notice your energy levels at different times of the day to determine your best time to exercise. By following your own body's schedule, you are more likely to follow your plan consistently.

7. Make your plan fit your life. Certain things in life are constants. You know that every day you will be involved with work, kids, and other activities. You will never stick to an exercise plan long term if it doesn't fit into your life.

8. Build a team. Everyone needs coaches and cheerleaders. Build a team of experts and friends who can support you. Your experts could be anyone from the owner of the vitamin shop to a personal trainer. You could also rely on expert resources, such as running and cycling magazines or even Internet websites. Using expert advice to educate yourself only solidifies the mental image of you as an athlete.

9. Get inspired. Inspiration can come from listening to certain songs or watching stories of people who triumphed over adversity. Being motivated and inspired to reach a goal can be like stoking a fire inside of you. I personally like watching *The Biggest Loser* to get inspired.

10. Be patient. Patience is a fruit of the Spirit and one thing that is necessary to reach any goal in life. Getting fit is no exception! Be patient with yourself if your progress is slower than you think it should be. If you keep going and don't quit, you will reach your goal.

Excuses No More

Have you ever been laying on the sofa and watching your favorite TV show when suddenly the actor starts running or playing a sport? And as you're laying there eating your bag of chips, you think to yourself, *I should go for a walk.* That's a fit-girl whisper!

When I was a fat girl, I used to hear that voice all the time. Whenever she whispered in my ear, the fat girl started her speech. She said, "Why bother? I'm so heavy that a walk wouldn't do me any good. It'd be like spilling a Dixie cup into the ocean." I thought for a minute or two and then agreed with the fat girl. So I continued to lie on the couch with potato-chip crumbs covering my chest. The fat girl had won another round in the battle of the bulge.

I also had to fight with the fat girl about going to the gym, especially when my skinny sister–in–law, who I talked about in the introduction, invited me to go with her every now and then. Just like I balked when she told me I should start a food journal, I balked at her invitations to the gym. Even while the fit girl considered the possibility—thinking it might be fun—the fat girl shook her head and whipped out a lengthy list of excuses that included why it was a bad idea. In particular, that fat girl reminded me that I didn't have cute clothes, people would probably make fun of me, and I wouldn't be able to keep up with my sister-in-law.

When I became a fit girl, do you know what I realized? My excuses were hogwash. First of all, it doesn't matter what you wear as long as your shoes are comfortable and won't cause blisters. That's all that matters. Before I started working out, I went to a specialty shoe store to have my feet properly fitted for a pair of shoes. I highly recommend you do the same. Your shoes don't necessarily have to be stylish, but they have to be a correct fit. As far as clothes, who wants to wear cute clothes? They'll just get sweaty and nasty. I wear shorts and a T-shirt, and I'm as comfortable as can be. After all, I'm there to work out, not be a sportswear model.

The second thing I discovered was most people are not thinking about you when they work out. They are typically in their own little world, consumed by their own routines, listening to their iPods, and concentrating on their form. That's how I am when I work out. I am usually so zoned in on what I'm doing that my friends literally have to grab my arm to get my attention. So the fat girl is wrong. No one is going to make fun of you. Quite frankly, no one really cares.

The third thing I realized is that you can keep up—with yourself, that is. When you are at the gym with a friend, don't fall into the trap of unhealthy competition. You have to do the best you can do at whatever fitness level you are at. Don't feel like you have to exercise like a triathlete when you step into a gym for the first time.

Is there something holding you back from exercising on a regular basis? Maybe you feel like you don't have enough time. I believe that if you make something a priority, you can make time for it. How many hours a day do you watch television? How many hours a day are you on the computer for nonwork related matters, like socializing on Facebook or browsing the Internet for stuff you probably don't need. Most of us take time to hang out with our girlfriends or spend hours chatting on the phone with friends.

Be honest with yourself. How much extra time do you spend doing things that are not a priority? I'm sure you can use that time to focus on improving your health. Now, I'm not saying you have to go to the gym every day. I'm just saying that if you want to be a fit girl, you're going to have to carve time out of your schedule to move your body.

I try to work out an hour a day at least four or five days a week. If that seems to be too much for you, think about it this way. Can you exercise for 30 minutes twice a day? What about 15 minutes four times a day? You can break this up by working out when you wake up in the morning, during your lunch break, and at the end of the day. Now doesn't that seem more reasonable?

If you have children and find yourself spending a lot of time driving your kids to soccer practice, art class, or dance lessons, try using the time you would spend waiting for them to take a brisk walk. You could even ask the other mothers to join you!

Guard Against Dehydration

When you start an exercise plan, you have to make sure you stay hydrated. To determine if you are drinking enough water, take your body weight, divide that number in half, and drink that much water in ounces. For example, if you weigh 200 pounds, you should drink 100 ounces of water every day. If you are active, staying adequately hydrated to avoid dehydration becomes even more necessary.

According to the American College of Emergency Physicians, in hot and humid conditions, an active person can become dehydrated in just 15 minutes. For a 130-pound person, losing as little as 1.3 pounds of fluid can lead to early fatigue and increase the risk of dehydration.

If you experience any of these symptoms, you may be dehydrated.

- dry lips and tongue
- a lack of energy
- muscle cramps
- bright-colored or dark yellow urine

If left untreated, dehydration can escalate to heat exhaustion or heat stroke and either can be deadly. The main symptoms for these include:

- fatigue
- dizziness
- nausea or vomiting
- headache
- rapid and shallow breathing
- high temperature
- rapid heart beat
- decreased alertness or complete loss of consciousness

If you experience these symptoms, doctors say you should stop activity immediately and cool down in the shade or an air-conditioned building. It's important to drink fluids to quickly replenish what you've lost through sweat.

Some tips to prevent dehydration and other heat-related illnesses include:

- Drink water before, during, and after exercise.
- If you exercise for more than an hour, drink a sports drink.
- Avoid caffeinated beverages and alcohol because even though they are liquids, these fluids dehydrate the body.
- Avoid carbonated beverages, which can cause bloating and keep you from drinking enough fluid to rehydrate.
- Wear light-colored, absorbent, loose-fitting clothing.
- Stay in cool, shaded areas when possible.

Ideas and Tips

Don't get too stressed about how to exercise and when. Just do it. The key is to activate your body. Move your body. Get up off the couch and do something physical. This could be yard work or something as simple as doing household chores. If you're not sure where to start, pick up a book about exercise at your local library or bookstore or talk to a trainer at a fitness club.

A good way to start moving is simply by walking. Walking doesn't require any special equipment or a gym membership. All it requires of you is to place one foot in front of the other and repeat.

Walking is great for your heart and lungs, and it also strengthens your leg muscles. If you walk briskly, you can burn approximately 300 to 400 calories in an hour, depending on your age and weight. If you have a significant other, walking is a great way to bond as a couple. There are a few couples in my neighborhood who walk together early in the morning. Some even use that time to pray.

Once you get into the habit of walking, I encourage you to challenge yourself and try to jog every couple of minutes. (Of course, talk to your doctor first and make sure he or she thinks it's a good idea based on your physical condition.) Keep things in perspective. Don't expect to a run a marathon quite yet. At first you might be able to only run from your mailbox to the one next door. That's okay. After a week or two, you'll probably be able to run from your mailbox to the one a couple doors down and then to the one a block over. Before you know it, you will be running a mile or more a day!

When Phillip and I were training for a half marathon, our coach recommended that we run for six minutes and walk for a minute. This method builds your endurance and makes it possible to run a longer distance. I have also been told that this run/walk method is great for weight loss because your heart rate rises when you are running and then slows back down when you are walking. This is called "interval training" and is what keeps your heart rate in the fat-burning zone.

Weight (or strength) training is another great form of exercise. When you build muscle, you burn fat. I know many women who are scared of bulking up. They think that if they work out with weights, they'll turn into the Incredible Hulk! While that's not physically possible because we don't have the high levels of testosterone that men do, I suggest starting out with lower weights and doing more repetitions. This will tone your muscles and make them long and lean. I try to stick with 10- to 15-pound dumbbells and perform 3 sets of 12 repetitions when I work out my arms, shoulders, and back. If you haven't been lifting weights, start out using lighter weights.

After we lost the weight, Phillip and I went to see a plastic surgeon. We were considering surgery to remove the extra skin around our midsections. You wouldn't believe the amount of excess skin that accumulates after you lose a hundred pounds! Our doctor told us we looked pretty good considering how much weight we'd lost. Our skin had sagged the least of anyone he had ever examined. He attributed it to the amount of exercise we had done and, in particular, weight training.

If you don't have a gym membership or don't have access to weights, there are many other ways you can get fit. You can replace dumbbells with common household items. All you really need is something with weight, right? Try lifting a full gallon of milk, large cans of vegetables, or even water bottles.

I routinely exercise in ways that don't involve any equipment at all. These are called "body weighted exercises" and include things like pushups, squats, lunges, and tricep dips. They actually use the weight of your body to tone your muscle. I also love using resistance bands because they are fun to use, and they are portable, so I can take them with me if I am traveling. Resistance bands can be purchased at any sporting goods store, and many even come with a DVD or instructional guide.

You don't have to dish out a lot of money to exercise. Take a trip to your local library. Many of them offer DVD rentals. Browse through the selection of fitness videos. Maybe they have *The Biggest Loser* DVDs. Rent a couple of different ones to see what kind of exercise regime you like. Try Pilates, yoga, or kickboxing. The best part is you can do these videos in the privacy of your own home!

You can also check out your local cable listings. FitTV is a great channel that provides many different forms of exercise, from ballet to weight training to boot camp classes to good old-fashioned aerobics. It's another way you can work out at home without spending a dime!

Here's another idea. Form a neighborhood fitness club. Invite a group of ladies to your house and try these videos with them. You might even want to start a walking club and take walks around the neighborhood. It's a fun way to socialize, activate your body, and form a support system of women who can encourage each other (and you) toward becoming a fit girl.

If you work outside of the home, talk to your coworkers about getting together before or after work to walk, run, or do an exercise video together. Here's a secret: Many employers want their employees to be healthy because it helps keep their insurance premiums down. You can get brownie points with your boss if you show interest in trying to save the company a couple of bucks. So take some initiative and get your fellow employees moving!

Consider joining a gym with your friends or coworkers. Many gyms offer a discounted group rate. Your company might even provide a discount at certain fitness clubs. Here's another idea: Instill healthy competition at work by organizing a contest to see who can spend the most hours working out per week or who can lose the most weight.

Galvanize your friends, coworkers, and neighbors by starting a "90-Day Fitness Challenge" with them. We know thousands of people who have done this and experienced incredible results!

These are just a few ways you can make exercise a priority in life. This thought bears repeating—don't get bogged down by what you do; just get moving!

Tips to Help You Stay Motivated

Part of the battle of starting an exercise plan and keeping with it is mental. It is important to get motivated and stay motivated! Here are some tips I've used or others have told me about to help you get started and keep going.

- Remind yourself about how good you will feel after a workout. Before you go to the gym, start talking to yourself about this good feeling. If you tell yourself it is going to be a positive experience, you will be more apt to believe it!

- Pamper yourself. Tell yourself this is "me" time. I love to put on my iPod and leave the rest of the world behind. It is a time to forget all my other troubles and focus on me. Like a massage or getting my nails done, working out is a form of pampering my body.

- It's all about the burn. When I work out, I like to wear a heart-rate monitor so I can keep track of how many calories I burn. Watching those calories add up helps me stay motivated because the more calories I burn the more weight I can lose!

- Think about how you are going to look. Visualize what you are going to wear as your body changes and you reach your goal. Let this visual picture motivate you.

- Read success stories. I find the success stories of others incredibly inspirational. If a fitness website has success stories, I'll almost always read them.

- Reward yourself! If you exercise for a few days, give yourself a reward. A week? Another reward. Everyone likes to get a prize when they have completed a goal. Make sure you reward yourself for a job well done!

- Fit into smaller clothes. Everyone has a pair of jeans in the back of the closet they want to fit into or a bikini that has never seen daylight. Get your "goal" clothes out and look at them and be inspired to keep going.

- Feel attractive. Everyone wants others to think they are attractive. If it motivates you to get that extra compliment from your husband or coworker, then use that to keep going.

- Enjoy the adrenaline rush. I find that after I run the first mile, I get a rush that helps me keep going. If I am struggling at the beginning of my workout, I tell myself to hang on because the adrenaline rush is coming soon.

- Get relief. When I have a particularly stressful day, exercise is a great way to relieve the tension. Exercise gives you an extra bonus because you are not only making your body healthier, but you are also removing the emotional strains of the day. Who doesn't like to multitask?

- Take time to contemplate. When I exercise, I make goals, think about things that I need to work on, and regroup. It is also a good time to pray and contemplate my spiritual walk.

- Join a group fitness class. Sign up for a class or boot camp—perhaps with a friend—and you'll be motivated to get there and work out. No one wants to be the member of the class who can't keep up, so it also makes you push beyond your comfort zone.

- Hire a coach or personal trainer. Not everyone can afford a personal trainer, but if you can, it is worth the investment. My personal trainer has been a coach, counselor, and trainer all in one. He pushes me beyond the limits I have set for myself, and that alone is motivating.

- Write it down. For some reason, writing down your exercise is extremely important. It is like climbing a mountain and looking over the valley when you get to the top. If you write it down for a week, you can look back on that week and celebrate your accomplishments.

- Take a "before" picture. It is a good idea to take a picture of yourself at the beginning of your journey to document your starting point. As you hit milestones, take more pictures so that you can see your progress. This is very motivating!

- Sign up for a race. Just sign up for one, and you'll be motivated to train. It can be a 5K walk or as long as a marathon, it doesn't matter. Having a goal motivates you to train harder.

- Avoid feeling bad or guilty for not exercising. I hate how I feel when I don't exercise, and so I remind myself of that to get up and get going.

- Live long enough to see your kids grow up and have kids. If you are obese, you know that losing weight is truly a matter of life and death. Use this knowledge to fuel your fire to work out.

- Step onto the scale. Weigh yourself once a week. As you see the numbers go down, you will be motivated to do more. There is no better feeling than losing unwanted weight.

- Reach a goal. Set a goal for your ideal weight, a waist measurement, a specific number of days to work out, or a number of miles to run in a week. Setting and tracking a goal help motivate you to complete that goal. Make it easily achievable.

- Post results on your social network. This is a great way to hold yourself accountable. If you tell all your friends that you are going to do something, you are more likely to do it.

- Read motivational quotes. Many Internet sites list a treasury of motivational quotes. Read them whenever you need a boost.

- Prepare for an upcoming reunion. The knowledge that you are going to see people you haven't seen in years is a great motivation.

- Plan a vacation or cruise. Knowing you are going to have to fit into a bathing suit and wear it in public is a great way to inspire change.

Common Challenges

I am asked many questions about obstacles women face regarding working out. The one that's most asked is how to fit exercise in when you travel for work or vacation.

I'll admit this can be a challenge, but it's not a challenge without a solution. Phillip and I know a lot about how hard it can be to exercise when you are hopping from one city to another, which is exactly what we did during our book tour for *The 90-Day Fitness Challenge*. For a long period of time, it seemed like every single day was packed with meetings, interviews, book signings, and red-eye flights. Some nights we slept as little as three hours. It was a busy season for us, and I didn't have much time to exercise. After a week of not working out, I started getting worried. I thought, *How can I be a fitness role model if I am not working out?*

I had to re-evaluate my situation. I looked at my schedule and analyzed where I could make some shifts. I noticed that I spent a lot of time sitting on my bottom while I was waiting to board planes. So if I had an hour to spare, instead of sitting at the gate, I walked around the terminal with my bags (as weight training). I also took advantage of being on my feet as often as possible. For instance, I took stairs instead of escalators and even walked to events (if the distance wasn't too great) instead of taking cabs.

Vacations can be problematic for many people. What do most people do during this time? Eat! As a fat girl, my vacations revolved around where we would eat and when. Now my mind-set has expanded. Vacations are no longer about restaurants, ice-cream parlors, and snacks. Vacations are now about swimming, running on the beach, hiking, and sightseeing on foot. I am not telling you not to eat out on vacation or enjoy delicious food; I'm just warning you not to make food a priority.

Instead, make activity a priority. Search for recreational activities you can do that involve moving around (like hiking). If you have children, run around the beach with them. Walk around amusement parks. Just get moving!

Boredom can be a challenge for folks who find themselves doing the same kind of exercises all the time. This happened to me. I did the same routine (walking/running on a treadmill and a certain weight-lifting regime) for a long time. When I got bored, I noticed that working out wasn't fun anymore. When it wasn't fun, I wasn't as motivated to do it.

As bored as I was, however, I was afraid of venturing out and trying different things. It required moving out of my comfort zone, and that was a rough thing for me to do! Taking a new class at the gym or trying a new sport intimidated the fat girl in me. Classes that involved rhythm or choreographed moves were even scarier. Here's the cool thing. I found that once I pushed myself to try new things—in spite of my fear—not only did I end up enjoying myself, but some of the new classes I tried quickly became my favorites! I would never know what types of fitness routines I like had I never given them a shot! Today I'll try anything at least once. The fit girl is not afraid to check out new cardio, swimming, spin, and even dance classes. When you get out of your comfort zone and explore new kinds of physical activities, you'll be surprised at how quickly your boredom goes away!

Retrain Your Brain

What are your specific challenges when it comes to exercise? Are you afraid (like I was)? Are you short on time? Are you unmotivated? Whatever has held you back from engaging in exercise as a fat girl is a thought process you have to overcome.

Making any type of change is a battle that begins in the mind. We all have certain belief systems regarding exercise, some of which were formed during childhood. When I was in elementary school, I remember having to complete fitness assessments. I tried as hard as I could to push myself, but I almost always finished last in all the competitions. I determined then that I was not athletic. This self-destroying belief continued on through middle school. I refused to put on my gym clothes and participate with the rest of the gym class on many days. Most of the time, I pretended I didn't feel well, but really I didn't want to be ridiculed for my lack of athletic ability by the other kids. I held on to that same mind-set in high school and in college.

It wasn't until I was 40 years old and on *The Biggest Loser* that I suddenly realized I was an athlete. Every fit girl is! I found out I was strong and could challenge myself physically in ways I never imagined before. I just had to retrain my brain from thinking I had no athletic ability to believing I did!

Maybe you are in a similar place. Maybe you were the kid who got picked last to play kickball. Maybe you have never felt like you were an athletic kind of girl. Let me remind you that your beliefs dictate what you are. If you believe it, it's true. So start believing good things! When you doubt yourself or allow fear to dominate what might be possible for you, you are believing a lie! I am not saying that it will be easy to whip your body into shape and become a strong and active fit girl, but it is possible! You can do it! I know you can, and I believe in you, fit girl!

Support! Support! Support!

If at all possible, find an accountability partner—someone who supports your fitness goals and believes in you. It's important. Whether that partner is a friend, a family member, or a personal trainer, having someone to challenge, motivate, and keep you from quitting is a great help.

My accountability partner is my trainer, DJ Jordan. I can't tell you how many times I worked out with him and felt tired, sick, sore, and even like my lungs were going to explode from how hard he worked me. It was during these times that he pushed me and coached me through the pain. He never let me quit.

I remember when DJ and I ran my first 5K race together. The race was called the "Midnight Flight" because it took place at night. Now, DJ was not a race novice. He had run many marathons and half marathons and could have easily run circles around me. When we stood at the starting line, I was petrified, and DJ could tell. He gave me a big hug and assured me, "Amy, you are going to be fine. I'll be right next to you the whole time." His presence was a huge comfort for me.

When we got to the halfway mark, we came to a big hill. This is when it started to get tough. I wanted to quit. But DJ would have none of it. He started talking to me about the finish line. He told me what it was like to go through the last stretch of the race. He said the course would be lined with people, and they would all cheer for me as I finished. He made me think about the goal, and his words helped me to keep going. I ran over the finish line to the sounds of people cheering. DJ was pointing at me and yelling to the crowds, "This is her first 5K!" It was a great moment—one I will never forget.

Who is your DJ? Who is your cheerleader? Who can hold you accountable to your goals and not let you throw in the towel? I am sure you can think of someone who would be willing to be that person for you. If you're not sure, pray that God will bring someone into your life to fill this role.

Make exercise a priority. It's a big part of being healthy, and I can promise you that you'll be glad you did. Now get up and move, fit girl!

The Importance of Sleep

Exercise is extremely important, but while we are starting our exercise program, we also need to keep in mind the importance of sleep. Make sure you get enough rest every night. Here is a list of some of the main reasons why sleep is so important.

- Learning and memory. Sleep helps the brain commit new information to memory through a process called "memory consolidation." In studies, people who'd slept after learning a task did better on tests later.

- Metabolism and weight. Chronic sleep deprivation may cause weight gain by affecting the way our bodies process and store carbohydrates and by altering levels of hormones that affect our appetite.

- Safety. Sleep debt contributes to a greater tendency to fall asleep during the daytime. These lapses may cause falls and mistakes, such as medical errors, air traffic mishaps, and road accidents.

- Mood. Sleep loss may result in irritability, impatience, inability to concentrate, and moodiness. Too little sleep can also leave you too tired to do the things you like to do.

- Cardiovascular health. Serious sleep disorders have been linked to hypertension, increased stress hormone levels, and irregular heartbeat.

- Disease. Sleep deprivation alters immune function, including the activity of the body's killer cells. Keeping up with sleep may also help fight cancer.

◈◈◈ Transformation Tips ◈◈◈

1. What fears have held you back from exercise? Were you the last kid picked in gym class? Do you associate working out with misery? Pray for strength to face those fears.

2. Think about your daily schedule. Can you find time to multi-task and get your workout done? Try doing something active while you wait for an appointment or parking your car farther away from the mall when you go shopping. Write down some ideas.

3. Who would make a good exercise accountability partner for you? Do you have a group of friends who would be willing to share this journey with you? Call one or two of them and start a fitness relationship.

4. Right now write down three ways to exercise that don't require a gym or special equipment. Can you tone your muscles with your purse or walk during your lunch break? Can you do some lunges while watching your favorite television show?

◈◈◈ Your Prayer ◈◈◈

Father, I pray that You would help me overcome my fears and excuses when it comes to exercise. Help me find creative and budget-conscious ways to move my body. Help me find someone who I can use as an accountability or support partner; someone who can encourage me to not give up. Thank You for giving me the strength I need to make my body healthy. Help me take care of this beautiful temple You have given me. In Jesus' name I pray. Amen.

Your Thoughts

Your Thoughts

You Can't Move Forward
If You Can't Forgive

*To forgive is to set a prisoner free and
discover that the prisoner was you.*

—LEWIS B. SMEDES

You know a little bit about my childhood, how I felt very alone, and how I tried to comfort my pain and fill the hole in my soul with food. In most movies, there is usually a particular sequence of events. A main character is faced with a conflict. This person goes through ups and downs to find the solution to her dilemma. Then, as if by magic, the character always finds a way out. Something happens—and poof—the problem that she was facing goes away. How I wish life was like that. I wish I could wave a magic wand over challenges, obstacles, and trials, say "Ta-da," and make them all go away. Unfortunately, life is more complicated.

It took a long time for me to heal and for my heart to become whole. I've found that we are complex beings with many layers. Being a whole fit girl doesn't usually happen instantly. There are usually several "ah-ha" moments when we stumble upon epiphanies and have the opportunity to change things about ourselves or our lives one piece at a time.

Throughout the years, I had built up walls and pushed down

emotions I didn't want to deal with. It was easier for me to numb myself by eating than to face the things that I had buried for so long. When those emotions and memories came flooding back, I learned one thing that set me free. It wasn't a magic or cookie-cutter solution. The key to unlocking those secret parts of my heart was forgiveness.

One of the most powerful ways to be set free from the fat girl and the deadly control of her vices is to forgive those who have hurt us. Only when the fat girl learns to forgive others—and even herself—is she able to fully transform into a fit girl.

Did you know that many times our addictions, including food, can be rooted in bitterness? When people hurt us or let us down, we have a tendency to get mad. And instead of forgiving that person and letting go of our anger, we hold on to our grudge like a security blanket. This bitterness causes a memory in our heart similar to a bruise. If someone stepped on your foot and you felt pain, you would naturally draw your foot back if that same person walked by you again. This is also true with your heart.

If your heart has been broken or neglected, you are probably going to avoid even the potential of future heartbreak at all costs. We are going to hide our heart and protect it from any pain. In the case of the fat girl, she will do this by eating herself silly. She will stuff her anger, pain, and bitterness in a tub of ice cream, a box of pizza, or a bag of donuts.

But the fit girl knows this is not the answer. The fit girl understands that only forgiveness can truly unchain a captive heart.

Are You Running Around in Circles?

I once heard a pastor teach a lesson on forgiveness. He related our lives to taking a vacation to a particular destination. Let's say you were going to Disney World, and while you were driving, you passed by your house a couple of times. Eventually (hopefully by the second time) you would realize that you were going around in circles. When you realized this, he said, you would stop and ask for directions or get a map and get on the right route to Disney World.

Many times forgiveness can be that map to changing the scenery in our lives. This pastor said if you are living your life and you see the same pattern repeatedly developing without making any progress, then maybe you need to ask God what the deal is. Obviously God is trying to get your attention, urge you to let go of some kind of hurt, and encourage you to move on.

I know that predicament well. On my way to becoming a fit girl, many of the issues I needed to deal with to move to the next level of my relationships, career, and even health involved forgiveness.

This reminds me of the nation of Israel. They wandered around the desert for 40 years because they didn't get that God would take care of them. Their past experiences were powerful enough to keep them chained to their past. Only when they began to let go of what had happened, were they able to walk into the Promised Land. Those Israelites had been slaves to the Egyptians for hundreds of years. They had been abused and treated like garbage by their captors. They knew they were God's chosen people, and yet they were living in shackles, bound by hard Egyptian rule.

I would bet that they felt abandoned by God at times. I am sure their experience made it difficult for them to believe they could ever be set free. But then something happened. God commanded Moses to be their leader and show them that freedom was possible. Moses performed many signs and wonders in front of the Pharaoh and demanded he let "God's people go." When the ruler finally agreed and the Israelites began their exodus toward the Promised Land, God continued to perform miracles for them. He parted the Red Sea. He gave them food every day. He even made water flow out of a rock so they would never be thirsty.

You'd think those signs and wonders would have strengthened their faith, but they didn't. Their former life as slaves had impaired their ability to trust God in spite of all of the miracles they had seen with their own eyes. Their pain and hurt had blinded them to the goodness of God. The Israelites walked around in circles in the desert for 40 years without arriving at the land God promised them not because they were lost, but because they didn't trust Him. In their lack of faith, the Israelites tried to do their own thing and made idols to other gods. They also tried to store up food for fear it would run out. They did everything in their own power to control their circumstances (sounds a lot like the fat girl in me).

When they finally got to the Promised Land, they saw giants there. These folks were so discouraged, they were ready to bolt. Surely God couldn't save them from giants. Finally Joshua and Caleb, two Israelite leaders who were great men of faith and believed in God's promises, convinced the people that God was more powerful than the giants that lived there. Joshua and Caleb weren't focused on the obstacles. Instead, they were focused on God. And you know what happened? Not long after, the Israelites finally set foot in the Promised Land.

What about you? Are you walking around in the desert? Do you keep seeing the same scenery over and over and feel like you aren't making any progress? Are you holding on to the past and not allowing God to work in your life today? If so, there just might be an area of unforgiveness in your heart that you have to deal with to move on and become a fit girl.

When Phillip and I had been married for about five years, we moved to Seattle, Washington, to help some friends start a church. It was the first time in my life I was far away from my family and in a city that was nothing like where I was from in South Carolina. It was a "desert" time for me. I believe that God needed to take me away from my comfort zone so I could deal with some of the things that kept me walking around in circles.

I remember being paralyzed by fear at times and afraid to go out of my house alone. I couldn't stand to look at myself in the mirror because I hated what I saw. I would wake up in the middle of the night from bad dreams about certain childhood memories I had tried to forget. Out of nowhere, I would experience uncontrollable bouts of sadness and felt unloved or unwanted. All of these things were keeping me from living a full and blessed life. Looking back at that period of time, I am convinced God took me there because He needed me to deal with those personal issues that were blocking me from my "promised land" and from becoming a fit girl.

people around her. The fit girl knows that we all have sinned and fallen short, so that is why she must show mercy to others.

Jesus is the perfect illustration of how to walk in forgiveness. He was the one who asked, "Why do you look at the speck of sawdust in your brother's eye and pay no attention to the plank in your own eye?… You hypocrite, first take the plank out of your own eye, and then you will see clearly to remove the speck from your brother's eye" (Matthew 7:3,5). Jesus was betrayed by His friends and by His disciples. He was beaten by His enemies and hung to die on a cross. After going through all of that, He asked His Father to forgive those who were killing Him by saying, "Father, forgive them, for they do not know what they do" (Luke 23:34). Wow! What a powerful example for us to follow.

I remember a time when my husband was involved in the real estate investment business. He would find a home that was a foreclosure or being sold at a really good price, buy it, fix it up, and resell it. During this time, he developed relationships with many subcontractors, vendors, and bankers to help him do business. We met a guy who had just started working as a banker at a local bank. He was close to our age, and we became friends with him and his wife.

After a few months, this guy brought up the idea that he and my husband should do an investment deal together. We thought it was a great idea. Phillip found a commercial property that he would remodel, and his friend would get the loan for the deal. Everything seemed to be going well until we found out that our banker worked out the loan in a way that wasn't exactly legal.

Since my husband's name was on the original paperwork, it initially seemed that we were a party to fraud. It also made the property impossible to sell. This was devastating for us because not only did it affect us financially, but we also lost our friends in the process.

Phillip and I felt very betrayed and angry. Our friend ended up facing grave legal issues, and he and his wife divorced. It was a very sad situation, and for a long time, bitterness festered in me. My husband forgave this man quicker than I was able to. Eventually, however, I realized that my anger wasn't hurting this man at all. It was a waste of my time, energy, and health. So I did what I knew I had to do. I forgave him. The anger went away and was replaced with compassion. I felt sympathy for his wife and kids. His poor decisions had damaged his life and the ones he loved. I can truly say with all my heart that I wish only the best for him and his family.

What does this have to do with fat girls and fit girls? When you hold on to bitterness and refuse to forgive, you are allowing the enemy to control your life. You are basically holding out your wrists and asking the devil to put handcuffs on you. Satan wants you to be in bondage so you can't live a full life.

Food addiction is bondage just like any other addiction. In order to have freedom in that area, you must be willing to forgive. The fat girl is in bondage; the fit girl is free. The fat girl holds on to bitterness; the fit girl lets it go. The fat girl hides in shame; the fit girl runs to God for forgiveness.

Perhaps you can't forgive someone because they have passed away. Maybe you were not able to have closure with them while they were still alive. If this is the case, it may be a good idea to write that person a letter. You could say all of the things in the letter that you never got to say to them while they were alive. You could read it out loud or take it to their grave site and read it there. This act can give you the closure you are seeking. This might also be helpful if you don't know where the person you need to forgive is (for instance, birth parents you've never met).

Forgiving Yourself

Many times the hardest person to forgive is yourself. Women from all over the country tell me they feel like such failures. It's a feeling that stems from many different reasons. Some women feel like failures because they aren't the perfect mother. Some of them feel like failures because they can't get control over some area of their lives. Some of them feel like failures because of something they did in the past. These women are constantly condemning themselves for one reason or another. It's an exhausting way to live!

Phillip and I were guests on a particular call-in radio show and were asked questions via email and phone about health and fitness. One lady emailed me her story. She related to my husband and me because she had a child who was diagnosed with cerebral palsy. She said that she and her husband had grieved over this diagnosis, and as a result, she had gained weight. She weighed over 300 pounds. She said that she would lose 20 pounds and gain back 20 plus more. Then she uttered these heartbreaking words, "I feel like such a failure."

I immediately thought, *How could this woman say that about herself?* This is someone who has had to deal with a challenge most people will never go through. While most mothers are scheduling play dates for their children, this woman is going to doctors and physical therapy appointments. While most mothers are dreaming about their child going to the Olympics or playing professional sports, this woman is wondering if her child will ever be able to walk.

This woman is living a hard life that most of us cannot even imagine. For her to say that she is a failure is an incredible statement. More importantly, it's a false statement. She is a perfect example of someone who needs to forgive herself.

I can relate to her experience. When Rhett was first diagnosed with autism, I constantly blamed myself. I felt guilty for eating too much seafood, painting baby furniture, and standing in front of the microwave while I was pregnant. I knew it must be my fault he had autism. If only I hadn't let him jump on the bed, he would not have hit his head that time. If only I had played with him more as a baby, his brain might have developed properly. If only I had rested more while I was pregnant, maybe he would have been normal.

Those thoughts kept me up most nights. What a waste of time! What-ifs, should-haves, and could-haves are pointless. You can't turn back the clock or rerun plays. You can't undo what's been done. It isn't my fault Rhett has autism, but even if it was, there is nothing I can do about it now. It took a long time for me to come to this realization.

The lady with a son with cerebral palsy needs to forgive herself and move on. She needs to be proud of the things she has been able to accomplish. She needs to realize that the strength that she is using to take care of her child is the same strength she can use to take care of her health. She needs to be able to forgive herself so she can begin taking better care of her spirit, mind, and body.

I heard the saying one time, "If the devil can't stop you, he will push you." It seems that one way he likes to push women is to make them focus on regrets. When you focus on the things you regret about your life, then you are always trying to do something to make up for the past. You always feel like you can't do enough to make up for your weaknesses.

Since we are not perfect beings, this process is about as productive as a person walking through quicksand. When you are in quicksand, the more you move, the deeper you sink. The more you focus on your regrets, the further behind you get. The fat girl wallows in self-pity and feels less than a person. The fit girl doesn't throw herself pity parties because she knows they don't produce anything good in her life.

A fit girl also focuses on her victories. She knows that when she forgives herself and thinks about the things she has done well, then she will have more confidence to conquer other giants in her life.

My husband and I love to sit and watch the Ironman competitions on television every year. These races consist of a 2.4-mile swim, a 112-mile bike ride, and a 26-mile run. Any one of those events would be challenging, but all three together is an incredible athletic feat. To make it even more brutal, all three events have to be finished in 15 hours. You have to be in tip-top shape to do that!

I especially love to watch the stories of the participants who compete after facing severe obstacles. Phillip and I will sit and cry (okay, maybe I'll be the only one crying) when we see folks running, swimming, or biking with prosthetic legs or amputated arms; people who have survived life-threatening illnesses, or senior citizens still running strong. These people are taking the obstacles in their lives, staring them right in the face, and overcoming them.

They had a choice. They could have sat at home and felt sorry for themselves, but they didn't. They opted to pick themselves up and do something rewarding and meaningful instead. Making this right choice embodies the spirit of the fit girl. She doesn't let the emotional weight in her life slow her down. She forgives herself and, like an iron-man (or woman), runs her life's race.

Have you felt the weight of something in your life holding you back? Do you feel like you are incapable of moving on because you can't forgive yourself for something? Or maybe you don't feel that you are worthy of God's forgiveness or love. I want you to know today that you are worthy. God made you, and you are His most valuable possession. You do not have to be perfect to earn God's love or approval. Jesus already did that for you. All you have to do is accept the forgiveness, grace, mercy, and love He freely offers to you.

To Forgive Is to Lose a Weight

When you forgive, you feel a million pounds lighter on the inside. When you hold things against other people or yourself, you literally feel weighed down in your heart. The Bible says in Isaiah 40:31, "But those who hope in the LORD will renew their strength. They will soar on wings like eagles; they will run and not grow weary, they will walk and not be faint." We are created to soar. If we don't forgive, we'll carry around extra baggage that makes it impossible to soar. Our spiritual wings will be clipped.

Let me share a story with you so you can see how a fit girl is transformed by forgiveness. A friend of mind was on a weight-loss journey at the same time I was. She had been estranged from her mother for years because her parents got a divorce when she was a teenager, and she blamed her mother for the split. Her mother had actually taken some of her sisters with her and left my friend to live with her father. This made my friend feel as though she was unloved. She was angry that her mother chose to split up their family. As an adult, one time she even told her mother that she was going to have to "love her from a distance," because she was still hurt by the fact that her mother left their family.

My friend did not speak to her mom for years. While she was try-ing to lose weight, her dad encouraged her to reach out to her mom and invite her to come along the health path she was on. At first my friend was reluctant, but eventually she realized it was a good idea. Her mother was delighted.

Taking the health journey with her mother forced her to confront all the bitterness that she held inside. When it got tough to face those emotions, all she wanted to do was run away. Instead, my friend made the decision to forgive her mother. The week she made this change, my friend told me that not only did she feel free in her heart, she had also lost six pounds! I'm not saying if you forgive someone, you'll lose weight. I'm just saying there is something spiritually and physically powerful about the act of forgiveness.

There is a medical reason for this. When we are stressed, our body produces the hormone cortisol. When released, this hormone causes us to hold on to weight, especially in the belly area. Holding on to bitterness, whether we realize it or not, is very stressful and can cause our body to release this hormone. I believe this is one of the reasons that many women carry extra weight in their midsection. True, we live in a stressful world. There are many things in this life that we cannot control, but we do have the choice to live a life of forgiveness.

When You Have to Forgive God

Did you ever think you might have to forgive God? It sounds crazy, doesn't it? But sometimes, when we don't have anyone to blame, it's convenient to blame Him when bad things happen in our lives. I know a woman who physically cannot have children. As a teenager, she was the neighborhood babysitter, and all the kids loved her. She wanted nothing more than to get married and have children of her own.

When she realized she was not going to be able to carry her own children, she immediately became angry with God. She thought it was cruel that God would give her the desire to have children but not the physical capability to have them. I encouraged her to think about adopting or other options.

Nothing I or anyone else said helped. She started drinking heavily. I wondered if perhaps this addiction was caused by the root of bitterness in her heart. I have a feeling it was. Eventually this woman got married to a man who had a son. I don't know if she has ever forgiven God for her medical issue, but I sure hope she has. It's a better way to live than the alternative.

⊙ TRANSFORMATION TIPS ⊙

If you are not sure how to forgive someone, the Bible offers us a tip. "Therefore I tell you, whatever you ask for in prayer, believe that you have received it, and it will be yours. And when you stand praying, if you hold anything against anyone, forgive him, so that your Father in heaven may forgive you your sins" (Mark 11:24-25). In other words, just do it.

Simply pray and believe that God will help you forgive whoever has hurt you. Trust Him to help you in this area. You don't have to wait for some kind of emotion to overtake you or wake up one day and magically be ready. Forgiveness is consciously deciding to release a person from guilt. It's as simple as that.

1. Identify any areas in your life where you feel as if you are repeating the same destructive pattern over and over. Are you in an abusive relationship? Do friends keep letting you down? Maybe you are stuck in a bad habit.

2. Pray and ask God to show you how to discover the cause of these destructive patterns. What can you do to change these behaviors? Do you need to forgive someone or ask them to forgive you? Let God show you who these people are.

3. Identify what you feel guilty about. Maybe you are condemning yourself for something you did in your past and are allowing it to consume your life. Maybe you are plagued by guilt because you feel like you've let people down. Write all these things down. Ask God to forgive you and help you forgive yourself for these things.

4. Name the people you can think of who may have hurt or wronged you. This may be a long list! Check your heart to make sure you have forgiven them. If not, do it now.

I admit that I've been angry with God a few times. Can you relate to this? You know those days when you can't figure out why this life takes an unexpected turn or why something didn't work out the way you thought it should.

One such time was actually during the finale of *The Biggest Loser*. I had worked so hard to win the "at home" prize. I felt like I had sacrificed everything to reach my goal, including time with my children and time at work. I thought that if I won the prize money, we would be able to pay off our bills and afford to take a vacation with our children.

Like many Americans, the economy took a toll on us. We had struggled financially ever since the real estate market took a downturn, and we even feared we would lose our home. This recession coincided with our season on the show, so winning that prize looked like the answer to all our problems. During the competition, there came a moment when I had to decide whether or not I was going to try for the highest percentage of weight loss. I decided to go for it, thinking that surely God would help me win. My children had sacrificed so much, and I wanted there to be some pot of gold at the end of the rainbow for them.

Sadly, that is not what happened. I lost the prize by four pounds despite my best efforts. Do you know how much those four pounds tormented me? I was happy for the girl who did win, but I felt as if my sacrifice was all for nothing.

At that moment I questioned why things happened this way and got a little upset with God. In retrospect I see that the fat girl was trying to take over my life again. I was acting like a spoiled little girl who wanted to control yet another situation. I was throwing a temper tantrum and expecting God to give me what I wanted. Of course, now I realize that He was trying to teach me how to deal with the fat girl once and for all. He wanted to show me that He was the one in control. I was facing a test that, sadly, I did not pass. So I had to ask God to forgive me, and I had to trust Him.

The Bible says in James 1:2-3 and 12, "Consider it pure joy, my brothers, whenever you face trials of many kinds, because you know that the testing of your faith develops perseverance… Blessed is the man who perseveres under trial, because when he has stood the test, he will receive the crown of life that God has promised to those who love him." Some tests involve forgiving yourself, others, and God. In order to become the fit girl who God wants you to be, you have to forgive.

Does this sound familiar? Have you ever had to release your anger and bitterness and forgive God or someone else? Sometimes this seems difficult to do. Why? Because when we hold on to our anger and don't forgive, somehow we feel like we are hurting the person that hurt us. The opposite is true. Living a life in which we can't forgive is like living a life with cancer. Bitterness will eat you up inside.

My husband and I met with a leader of World Vision, a wonderful Christian organization. He was telling us a story about some of the work they had done in villages all over the world. He explained that they go to a village and assess the way they can have the most positive impact on that particular area. He told us about was a village where the inhabitants were getting sick because their water source was contaminated. Apparently the water for the village came from a spring at the top of a high mountain. Because the spring was not covered, animals came and drank out of it. They discovered that a cow had come to drink from the spring, had fallen in, and died. This one animal contaminated the water for a whole village! The World Vision staff covered the spring and ran a pipe from the spring to the village to protect the water. Doing this kept the poison from getting into the water.

This reminds me of what one root of bitterness can do to our hearts if we don't dig it out. The Bible says in Luke 6:45 (NLT), "A good person produces good things from the treasury of a good heart, and an evil person produces evil things from the treasury of an evil heart. What you say flows from what is in your heart." The fit girl knows that she must guard her heart from things that contaminate it. Like the World Vision workers covering the water source, we must take measures to keep our heart free from bitterness. In Proverbs 4:23 (NLT), the Bible says, "Guard your heart above all else, for it determines the course of your life." If our hearts motivate and affect everything we do, then it is pretty important that we don't let anything poison it. We must quickly forgive if we want to be free. If you are keeping anything in your heart that is holding you back, then release it today. Let the fit girl take over!

❦ Your Prayer ❦

Dear Lord, thank You first and foremost for the forgiveness You gave when You sent Your Son to die for us. Thank You that by the blood of Jesus, I am saved, delivered, and healed. Please look at my heart and search out any unforgiveness or bitterness I may be harboring. If there is something I need to let go of, open my eyes and reveal it to me. Forgive me where I have wronged others. Forgive me for letting those things consume me. Help me forgive where I need to. And thank You for Your mercy and grace. Teach me to live forgiveness, grace, and mercy as You have bestowed them on me. In Jesus' name I pray. Amen.

Your Thoughts

Your Thoughts

Embrace Your Uniqueness

*As we grow as unique persons, we learn
to respect the uniqueness of others.*

—Robert H. Schuller

When I was a teenager, I hung out with a group of one-of-a kind individuals. We weren't bad or wild kids, but we were a little different. We were proud of the fact that we were nonconformists. We wore crazy clothes, listened to alternative music, and some of us even dyed our hair. I once dyed my hair orange and shaved it on one side, leaving the other side long.

I appreciated my friends because we danced to the beat of a different drum. We were a group of misfits, and we loved each other for the fact that we were different and didn't care what anyone thought about us. We embraced—even celebrated—our uniqueness. To this day, I look back on those times with fondness. I like thinking about a bunch of crazy teenagers who knew and appreciated the uniqueness with which they were created. Sadly, this is a challenge for many Christians today. We don't want to be different. We want to be just like everyone else.

As I grew older, I evolved and let my hair grow out to its natural color (until I realized that blondes have more fun). But one thing never changed. I often felt as though I was a little different. Usually I was okay with that, but sometimes there were times when I desperately wanted to be like someone else. When the pressures of other people, society, or even my own insecurities became too much for me, I would feel guilty for not being someone other than me.

I agonized over the things that came so naturally for other people; things like cooking a nice dinner for my family. When my husband and I were going to Bible school, my grandfather came to visit us. I wanted to impress him with my cooking skills and decided to make vegetable beef soup and corn bread. I had made it before without any notable disasters, so I felt it would be pretty safe to do it again.

This time, though, I cooked the meal on high, and it burned and stuck to the pan. Instead of leaving the stuck part to the bottom of the pan, I thought I could improvise. I had the brilliant idea of scraping up the burnt layer and stirring it into the soup. So instead of it just tasting a little burnt, it also had chunks of the burnt residue floating in the soup. Back then we rarely bought ground beef because it was too expensive, and so I was in tears. I failed at cooking the perfect meal and wasted money we didn't have.

My grandfather was so sweet and assured me that he loved things that were a little burnt and told me we could eat it just like it was. Still, we all knew the truth—it tasted horrible! I could barely eat two bites, but my grandfather ate the whole bowlful. He blew me away when he asked for a second helping. It was such a sweet gesture, but there was no hiding the fact that I wasn't Julia Childs.

After I had my first child, I remember desperately wishing I could be like some of the super moms who I thought had it all together. In my mind, they were professional mothers. They would put their child down for a nap at the same time every day and had them on a strict feeding schedule. It seemed like their children's clothes were always clean, they behaved tantrum-free in public, and they were enrolled in every sport, club, or group available.

This was quite a difference from my mothering style. I randomly shoved a bottle or goldfish crackers into my son's mouth when he cried.

I strapped him in his car seat and went for a ride to get him to sleep. I also chose the color of my clothes to blend in with baby food colors, since I wore more of my boy's food on my clothes than he swallowed.

Many times I tried to work from home or my car as an interior designer. I bet if I asked my now 15-year-old son the difference between chintz and pin-tucked silk, he could tell you because he spent so many hours in fabric shops. Needless to say, I did not win any mother-of-the-year awards. The funny thing is that my kids survived and actually have turned out pretty well (so far) in spite of what I thought was less-than-perfect parenting skills. My boys are polite and tolerant, and each of them is blessed with unique and wonderful qualities. No, I haven't been the perfect parent, but I tell you what, I have raised some great kids.

Fat-Girl Thinking

Here's the thing. The fat girl has a problem embracing her own uniqueness. She typically focuses on what she lacks, what others have that she wishes she had, or what she thinks would make her better if she had it—a skinny body, clear skin, a big bank account, or a hot husband. Oftentimes this takes the shape of comparing herself to others. This is especially challenging for me and, I believe, for women in general.

I have always had thin, stringy hair. Anytime I see a girl with long, thick hair, I get the worst case of hair envy. I have even perused the aisles of beauty supply stores looking at hair extensions and wondering if I could benefit from them. I'm also not fond of my long, big nose. I remember watching the TV show *Bewitched* as a teenager and thinking that I would never conjure up any spells with my big honker. The main character, Samantha, had the cutest little button nose and was so adorable when she would crinkle it up and do her spells.

I can keep going. I have this one group of friends that I affectionately call the "supermodels." If you saw them, you would understand why. Each one is a size zero or two, and they all have long, beautiful hair. They are always dressed to the nines in the latest fashions. They know how to apply their makeup like a professional makeup artist.

One of these friends asked my husband and me to be in a fashion show for a charity event. I had never felt so insecure in my life. For starters, you have to know how to walk down the runway, stop and pose, turn, and then walk back up the runway. You have to master the art of "the walk" with grace and a sultry look on your face. I'll admit that I am not the most graceful person, especially in heels. I am clumsy and have been known to trip over my own feet. So when I hit that runway, I felt like I stuck out like a sore thumb.

Now I am not saying I am hideous to look at or that I don't know how to walk, but when you compared me to the supermodels, it was evident they were more equipped to do this kind of thing than I was. God had given them a grace and poise that He clearly did not think I would need to fulfill my purpose in life. They were meant to do this stuff; I wasn't.

Fit Girls Work with What They Have

Though I have admitted some of my insecurities, I want you to know that I try very hard not to compare myself to other people when it comes to the way I look. We all have things about us that are beautiful, and it's great to be able to focus on what they are. I try to accentuate the positive and minimize the negative. For instance, I love my eyes. I think they're very pretty. This is why I try to make them stand out as the focal point on my face.

The same thing is true with our bodies. I believe that it is so important to exercise and try to keep in shape, but all of us have areas that look better than others. I feel like my arms, shoulders, and legs look pretty good, but my stomach and bottom not so much. So when I dress, I try to find clothes that show off my better features. That's why you will often find me wearing a halter top in the summer. I am trying to draw attention away from the areas that I'm not so excited about. You probably feel like you have body parts that aren't as good as others. It's okay. We all do!

When I was a teenager, I told my dad one time that I thought I was ugly. First, he reassured me that I was beautiful. Second, he told me a story about a particular actress, who at the time was considered to be the hottest sex symbol alive. He had heard her say in an interview that as a teenager she was considered an ugly duckling. Back in the day, she was too skinny, wore braces, and the boys in her class always teased her. I could hardly believe that what he was saying could be true. This movie star was the epitome of beauty, and she thought she was an ugly duckling? But the story did bring some peace to my mind because I realized that even the most beautiful person can have moments of insecurity.

My husband tells a story about when he worked out alongside a top fitness trainer and weight-loss expert. They had gone to a boutique-style gym in West Hollywood to do a boot camp class together. At the time, Phillip was a hundred pounds overweight, and he was having a tough time in the class. He looked over at this woman to see how she was doing, and to his surprise, she was having a tough time as well!

Phillip said this was an "a-ha" moment for him. If this world-class trainer was struggling through the workout, then he must be stronger than he thought. He was doing the same workout that she was doing, plus he had an extra hundred pounds on his body. Though he struggled, he was still able to finish the class!

You see, you can never put someone else on a pedestal and put yourself down. We are all human, and we all have struggles, challenges, and issues with self-confidence. Don't focus on other people's strengths to the point you ignore your own.

Fit Girls Stop Focusing on Their Flaws and Start Focusing on Helping Others

When we focus on comparing ourselves with others, it makes us self-centered instead of other-centered. If we are always worrying about the things we don't have or thinking about our flaws, we won't recognize the needs of those around us or consider what we could possibly do to help them.

This reminds me of a woman I went to church with once. I heard from several people that she was a talented artist. I saw her at church every

Sunday, and as soon as she walked into the building, it was as if a dark cloud came in with her. She walked with her head dropped down and never looked at anyone in the eye. If you ever stepped out to talk to her, all she ever talked about was the trouble in her life. It got to the point that I actually started avoiding her because even if I was in the greatest mood, I felt as if a wet blanket had been thrown on me after talking to her.

I know that others felt the same way. It became a bad pattern because the less people talked to her, the more it reinforced her belief that she wasn't good enough. The crazy thing was she was the one pushing people away by being so negative all the time.

Imagine if this same woman stopped feeling inferior and started valuing herself and the talents God blessed her with. She could have thought of ways to use her gifts to help someone else. Maybe she could have taught art to children or painted a mural for the church. If she hadn't been so focused on herself and, instead, was able to give in to other people's lives, she might have found more joy in living.

What Fit Girls Know

Let me tell you some things about fit girls. They

- recognize and use their gifts.
- recognize that God has given them a specific purpose for their lives.
- recognize that God has given them exactly what they need to fulfill that purpose.
- value their unique and special qualities, even if others think they are different.

It is important for the fit girl to recognize the gifts that God has given her. Some of us are so busy looking at other people and what they have that we forget to examine what God has gifted us with. You may think that you do not have any talents or unique qualities, but think about what you are passionate about. What do you love to do more than anything in the world? Do you love working with children, making things with your hands, or encouraging people? Your deepest desires hold a clue to the gifts that are uniquely yours.

Often we think that the gifts and talents we are gifted with come so naturally to us that *everyone* has and makes use of them. Here's an example. I know someone who loves to do taxes. It's like a game for her to uncover the most deductions and come up with the best refund she can for her clients. When I think about anything involving accounting or numbers, I get an instant headache. Who in the world would ever choose accounting as a profession? But she absolutely loves it! Why? Because God has given her a gift for it.

For myself, I have always loved everything to do with interior design. As a child, I could spend hours coloring with a big box of crayons and was fascinated by what colors looked like on paper. I would also take different shapes of wooden blocks and create floor plans with them. If you give me a paint fan, fabric swatches, window treatments, and mismatched furniture, I can put together a beautiful room in no time. It comes naturally for me. But you know what? I have friends who labor for months over what color to paint their bedroom. It's hard for them! If we take a minute to look at what brings us joy, it's probably an indication of what God has created us to do.

Years ago I worked with a girl who told me about a dream she had. She said that in her dream she was walking with Jesus in a house that had many rooms and doors. When they came to a door, they opened it up and stepped into a room filled with gifts of all different shapes and sizes. The deeper they ventured into the house, the more beautiful and ornate the packages were in the rooms. They finally came to the last room, and the gifts were breathtakingly beautiful. My friend asked Jesus, "Who are these gifts for?" He answered, "These gifts are placed in My people. Anyone who is willing to trust Me with the plan I have for their life will find them."

When she told me that dream, I got chills. Sometimes we have dreams because we have eaten too much pizza, and sometimes we have dreams because God has a specific message to give to us. I believe that was a dream from God.

Have you ever seen a beautiful quilt? My great-grandmothers on both of my parents' sides used to make them. I snuggled up with one every night and would wonder about the different fabrics as I fell asleep. As a little girl, Mom sometimes told me the stories behind each of those scraps of fabric. Some of them were expensive and some of them were from flour sacks. Some brought back memories because they were taken from dresses she wore as a child or from her grandfather's overalls. Some were brightly colored while others were light pastels. They were all different and came from different places. Some of the fabrics on their own weren't very special, but when they were sewn together with all of the others into the quilt, they became a beautiful work of art. We are God's "pieces of fabric." We may look fairly plain on the outside, but when we are doing the purpose that God created us for, we become beautiful and special. The Bible says in Ephesians 2:10, "For we are God's workmanship, created in Christ Jesus to do good works, which God prepared in advance for us to do." He has created us for a specific purpose and equipped us with gifts to fulfill that purpose. We are unique for a reason.

I once heard a preacher by the name of Miles Monroe speak at a church. He said something that struck me so powerfully that I have carried it with me ever since. He said that graveyards were sad places not just because of the lives lost but because of the wasted potential. He went on to say that graveyards are places that are full of songs that were never sung, books that were never written, and dreams that never came to pass. This, he said, is the true tragedy of death.

How often do we waste our time and potential comparing ourselves to others, longing for their qualities, and, in the meantime, overlooking the many special qualities God has given us? I wonder what wonderful paths God could take us down if we only recognized and used the talents He gave us to fulfill His purpose for our lives?

What legacy will your life leave? What gifts that God has placed inside you will go unused? A few years ago, I had the opportunity to be a guest on *The Oprah Show*. Hung on the wall in one of the backstage rooms was this quote from George Bernard Shaw's *Man and Superman*: "This is the true joy in life, the being used for a purpose recognized by yourself as a mighty one; the being thoroughly worn out before you are thrown on the scrap heap; the being a force of Nature instead of a feverish selfish little clod of ailments and grievances complaining that the world will not devote itself to making you happy."

This quote spoke to me. I believe that God wants us to be completely used up when we die. I want to be wrung out like a wet dishcloth with not one bit of potential left in me. Do you want that for your life? Then embrace your uniqueness.

Fit girls also recognize that they were created for a specific purpose. They are always working on what they were created to do—whether it's being a great mother, a business owner, a teacher, or something else. In lesson one, I talked about the empty hole in our soul that only God can fill. God gives us the Holy Spirit—the ultimate gift—so that He can fulfill His purpose in this world through us.

I can't say this enough. You have a unique mission. If you are busy looking at what other people have and what you don't, you might miss out on doing what only you can do. You might miss out on doing the thing that you were created by God to do.

This reinforces my belief that God has created us and equipped us with everything we need to fulfill our destiny. If we do the best we can with what God has given us, He will take care of the rest. I believe the reason we don't have some gifts or talents that others have is because we don't need them. God has only given us that which we need.

I like to think about my children when I ponder this truth. They are always asking me for something that I know they don't need, like a gadget, toy, or video game. "But, Mom," they always complain, "I just *have* to have it!" My children are masters in the art of persuasion when it comes to trying to get what they want. They will try to convince me that the thing will make their lives complete. But as their mother, I know what they really need and what they don't need. In fact, if they don't get it after a few days, most likely they won't even remember asking me for it!

However, when I sense the object encourages a God-given gift or talent, I am excited to give it to them when they ask. For example, my middle son, Pearson, received a cheap guitar as a gift and started teaching himself how to play it. He learned so many songs so quickly and had such a passion for music that I sensed he might have a gifting. When he asked for a really nice guitar and a keyboard for Christmas, I knew this was something that would ultimately serve his purpose. I felt like it might help him fulfill a desire God had placed in him. Today he is using those instruments to make instructional videos to teach people how to play them. He even puts these videos on the Internet. I would say that buying him that guitar and keyboard was a wise investment.

Fit girls also appreciate and value their unique and special qualities, even if others see them as being different. Let me tell you a story about a little boy. This little boy seemed to always be in his own world. At school it was hard for him to pay attention in class, and he had trouble learning in the same way his classmates did. This boy's teacher expressed her concerns to his mother and suggested that something may be wrong with him. The teacher even called the boy uneducable.

This boy was only in the first grade, and his mother made a decision to homeschool him. Surprisingly, she discovered that her little boy could learn. Not only could he learn, but today is known as one of the greatest geniuses ever born. This little boy was Thomas Edison, one of the greatest inventors (over 1000 inventions!) of all time. If he hadn't fulfilled his purpose, we might not have the lightbulb, rubber tires, or communication as we know it. I wonder if maybe the geniuses of our world are touched with being a little abnormal so that they can think outside the box and do whatever unique task God has planned for them.

It always encourages me when I hear this story because it reminds me of my son Rhett. Right before Rhett was officially diagnosed with autism, I knew there was something a little different about him. He was withdrawn, and it was hard to get and keep his attention. About the same time I read the story about Thomas Edison, we found out that Rhett was autistic. Even though Rhett has disabilities and limitations, he has other abilities that are unique only to him. Who knows what God has planned for my little boy? All I know is that God has a way of using people who are different to do great things.

When I look back at the paths my life has taken, I marvel at God and His mysterious plan. I had clues in my heart about what my future might hold, but I never could have guessed the road map God would use to get me there. I knew, for example, that I was called to the ministry when I was in my early twenties. I went to Bible school, and at first I thought I was supposed to be a missionary. I tried to raise support to go to the mission field, but something didn't feel right. Instead, my husband and I took over a youth ministry at a small church.

This was a wonderful time in our lives, and we saw God use us to bless many young people, though we were never able to do it full-time. Next, we helped plant a church in Washington State but were only there for a short time before we decided to move back to South Carolina. By this time, we were frustrated by trying to be full-time ministers, so we decided to go into business for ourselves.

It was great for a season, but as the Bible says, "The gifts and the calling of God are irrevocable" (Romans 11:29 NKJV). Who would have ever thought that two people who had ballooned to obesity would be used by God to have a ministry through weight loss? This just shows you that everyone has a unique path to walk. Trying to be like someone else can keep you from following the path God has specifically designed for you.

Your Turn

Take a few moments to think about your own life. Do you often feel sad because you can't do or don't have something? Try turning your thought processes around and thinking about the things you can do and the things you do have! Count your blessings rather than your deficiencies, and you will see the world through a more positive life. Become a "glass half full" person rather than a "glass half empty" one. It will make all the difference in the way you view the world.

In an article from the *Wall Street Journal* health blog, dated March 29, 2010, author Shirley S. Wang asks the question, "Can food be addictive?" She answers this question with a study published in *Nature Neuroscience*. This study was trying to prove whether or not the same changes in brain pathways developed with compulsive eating as did with drug addiction.

The study was conducted on rats that were fed high-calorie foods. As they ate and became obese, the parts of the brain associated with pleasure began responding in the same way they would if they were activated by cocaine or heroin. Rats who didn't have access to the junk foods didn't exhibit the same brain changes in the dopamine receptors. Even after the rats that were given the junk food no longer had access to it, the brain changes persisted.

"The results of this study could provide insight into a mechanism for obesity," Paul Kenny, an author on the study and professor at Scripps Research Institute, said in a statement. "It's possible that drugs developed to treat addiction may also benefit people who are habitual overeaters."

Loving yourself for who you are enables you to give yourself a break and relax. When we relax, we are better equipped to hear the Holy Spirit. When we are lead by the Holy Spirit, then we can make the right choices and decisions.

Don't play the compare game. It will only bring you anxiety and depression. You will become like a hamster on a wheel, always striving toward something but never making it. Don't live your life trying to fit into a mold that God never created you to fit into. Appreciate the mold He made you from! Do focus on your strengths. Do focus on your giftings. Do focus on how God made you unique.

The Bible says that we are fearfully and wonderfully made (see Psalm 139:14). When I think of the word "fearfully" in this sentence, I think about the first time I saw Mount Rainier, a huge, snow-capped mountain near Seattle. It is often hidden by clouds because it rains most days. On a clear day, however, the mountain is visible and breathtaking. When I saw it for the first time, I was a little afraid and awestruck at its beauty.

I think that God looks at us, His creation, like that. He made us each with a special gift that will take everyone's breath away when that gift is revealed. I also believe that one way that God is expressed through us is when we use our gifts to glorify Him.

The fit girl is aware of all of these things and is thankful to God for the unique way He made her. She goes after her dreams because she knows that God has placed them there and will guide her until they are fulfilled, no matter how crooked the path may seem at times. The fit girl is aware that His plan is perfect, and she trusts Him to guide her steps.

We have all been gifted with different talents and different purposes. We all have different road maps on the inside of us. God has a plan for your life that only you can do! So embrace your uniqueness, fit girl, and be proud of how wonderful and unique God made you!

❧ TRANSFORMATION TIPS ❧

1. Look at yourself in the mirror and write down all of the things you like about yourself. Then write down all the unique qualities you have. Write down things that you are good at. Don't leave anything out. If you won the fifth-grade spelling bee, write it down. If you nursed a friend back to health, write it down. Keep this with you to be reminded of how special you are.

2. Keep a dream journal. In it, write down all the things you would like to do with your life. Be specific in what you write. Maybe it's taking a dance class, learning to speak another language, or riding a motorcycle. Write down any desire in your heart that jumps out at you. Writing things down is important because it makes your ideas real. Studies have shown that you are likely to achieve written goals rather than ideas you keep only in your head. Before you know it, you will be marking things off the list!

3. Write down the names of three people you admire. They could be people you know or historical or biblical figures. Do some homework. Find out what their struggles or challenge have been. When you discover that they are just as human as you and that they had their own set of flaws and insecurities, it will help you feel a little more confident. It will help you put your own insecurities in perspective.

4. Reflect on your life. Have you ever been disappointed that something didn't quite work out the way you wanted it to, later see the situation within the big picture, and were thankful that one thing didn't work out? Write down those moments and appreciate the plan God has for you.

Your Prayer

Father, thank You for the way You made me. I am thankful that You made me for a unique purpose and plan. I ask that You reveal to me the things You want me to do with my life. I ask You to help me not compare myself to others but help me appreciate the ways that You made me special. I ask for Your hand to be on my life as I follow after the unique plan You have for me. In Jesus' name I pray. Amen.

Your Thoughts

Focus on Others

*I am a little pencil in the hand of a writing God
who is sending a love letter to the world.*

—Mother Teresa (Agnes Gonxha Bojarhiu)

Becoming a fit girl is all about focusing on the right things. What you focus on tends to expand. If you are constantly focusing on cheeseburgers, then all you are going to want to do is eat cheeseburgers. If you focus on your flaws or things you don't like about yourself, then all you are going to do is stress out about those things. If you always focus on your agenda or your own little world, you will be too self-absorbed to see people you could bless.

When we live our lives self-centered and not other-centered, we are not truly "fit" in all the ways God wants us to be. We need to be fit from the inside out. One way to do this is to acknowledge our blessings and figure out ways we can use them to help those around us. We all have a gift or talent God has given us to meet someone else's need. When we help others this way, we are living the kind of life God has called each and every one of us to live.

This truth applies to the fat girl too. As a fat girl, you can be so self-conscious that you are always thinking about yourself. You waste so much time and energy worrying about how other people see you or feel about you, that you can't think about anyone or anything else. As a fat girl, you can also become so obsessed with losing weight that you take drastic and unhealthy measures to try to get the weight off.

Being intensely focused on any one area of your life is not healthy. Life is about balance. When you become a fit girl, you are free to live without the particular worries that once plagued the fat girl. This gives you the room to think about the needs of others. Too many people are struggling with the fat-girl mentality. Once you have transformed into a fit girl, you can help others do the same thing! Isn't that something to look forward to?

We can choose to wear positive glasses or negative ones. I want to encourage you to put on and look through the positive shades. That way you will be able to see how you can make a difference in the world by helping others.

The Problem with Our Problems

When you are going through challenges, it is so easy to pray that God would bless just you or your family. It can be tempting to minimize prayer to something that goes like this, "Bless us four and no more." This is true even when you are struggling to lose weight. It's because our natural tendency is to be selfish and only concerned about our own needs.

It's normal to get so wrapped up in your own struggles that you can't be compassionate toward anyone else. When Rhett was diagnosed with autism, all I could think about was how much of a problem his disability was. I know for a fact that during that time, there were members of my family and some of my friends who were dealing with pretty serious issues of their own. Those negative glasses I was wearing made it impossible to see anyone else's problems.

Instead of being a good sister, daughter, or friend, I felt sorry for myself and constantly bemoaned my problems. My husband was struggling with his business, but instead of supporting him, all I could do was blame him for everything bad that was happening. My circumstances seemed so big because I had simply allowed myself to focus only on them. Nothing else existed for me. No one else had problems as big as mine. I found myself in a never-ending pity party.

When God finally put me in my place with my son, it caused me to shift my focus. I finally realized how selfish I had been. I came to understand how I had alienated members of my family because I was huddled in a corner with my own problems. I realized that I hadn't been there for my friends when they needed me. I didn't have time because I was stuck feeling sorry for myself. I also figured out that when all my attention was given only to my obstacles, I had completely ignored the wonderful things about my son and how he blessed our family.

10 Ways You Can Help Your Community in 30 Minutes or Less

1. Carry a garbage bag while walking through the neighborhood and pick up litter along the way. As a by-product, you can fit some exercise into your day.

2. Shop with locally owned businesses, saving time and money. Many locally owned businesses offer services like free gift wrapping and delivery, and a percentage of your sales tax goes directly to the local community.

3. Find positive aspects of your community and share them with other people. A positive image encourages residents to shop locally, increases the chance new businesses will open in the area, and promotes growth.

4. Attend a local festival or other event. Many have free admission and activities. Most festivals are actually fund-raisers for nonprofit organizations that make their money through sponsorships. Since sponsors look at attendance numbers to decide how much to give, your family can add to the number and help increase what businesses give next year.

5. Write a letter to local elected officials and encourage them to make good decisions for the community. People work harder when they know they are appreciated. Elected officials seldom hear enough encouraging words.

6. Put a potted plant on your front porch. When your home looks spruced up, it makes the whole neighborhood and the community look better.

7. Take dinner to an elderly neighbor. If you have a family of four, cook enough dinner for five one night and deliver a plate to the widow next door. Your delivery helps you to get to know your neighbors better. Police promote knowing your neighbors as the best way to fight neighborhood crime.

8. Look for opportunities to give in your community. Many schools collect items, such as canned foods, old coats, toys, and eyeglasses, for less fortunate families.

9. Vote. While the presidential election comes around only once every four years, elections happen every year. Check out the candidates for local and state elections.

10. Encourage your employer to sponsor local events, join a civic organization, or allow employees to volunteer during work hours. Many businesses have volunteer programs to reward employees for volunteering. Local news media often cover large volunteer events, and having employee representation gives businesses extra publicity.

Recently I went to an event at Rhett's school where they were giving out a bunch of awards. As I sat in the audience looking at the sea of children waiting to see if they would receive an award, I was suddenly struck with an epiphany. Of all the kids in that room, I realized that there was no kid I would rather call mine than Rhett. And I'm not saying that for dramatic effect either.

I really knew that he was my favorite little guy in the room. You see, out of all the children there that day, Rhett was the life of the party. He was smiling, laughing, and waving wildly at me. He was drawing a lot of attention to himself, but he didn't care one bit about what anyone thought about him. He was completely free and happy. I looked around and noticed that he was making everyone smile. His enthusiasm was contagious. (The name "Rhett" actually means enthusiastic, and it is so fitting for him.)

All the teachers hugged Rhett as they walked by. The other kids patted him on the back as he came near them. No one was a stranger to him that day. He was full of joy and positive energy and in that moment—the way we all should be. I realized why I love him so much and how very blessed I am. You know what else? My son made the honor roll. When his name was called, he ran up to the stage and danced a little dance for everyone! Everyone laughed, and he was tickled pink to be the center of attention.

What if I had always looked at Rhett's disability as a problem and defined him by that his whole life? What if I couldn't focus on the blessing that he is? I would have cheated myself out of so much joy. I would have also missed out on many opportunities to help those who have autistic children of their own. I wouldn't have had the life experience that I now use to bring comfort and educate other parents.

20 Community Organizations That Could Use Your Help

1. Homeless shelters
2. Food banks
3. Letters to Soldiers
4. Ronald McDonald House
5. Special Olympics
6. Habitat for Humanity
7. State parks
8. City programs
9. Helping Others Learn to Read
10. Hospitals
11. Libraries
12. Senior citizens centers
13. Animal shelters
14. United Way
15. Red Cross
16. Salvation Army
17. Environmental organizations
18. Political campaigns
19. Local schools
20. Website creation

What's Possible When We Look Outside of Ourselves?

I remember a sweet young lady who came to one of our first 90-Day Fitness Challenge events. She was going through the initial stages of having her son diagnosed with autism and had a similar story to mine. This woman had turned to food to comfort herself during this time. When she introduced herself to me, she was in tears. When I looked into her eyes, I saw myself a few years earlier.

I understood the pain she was going through. Meeting her took me back to that dark season, but it also made me feel really blessed to be on the other side. I was able to comfort her with hope and confidence because I had gone through the same thing. I shared with her that she was probably walking through the hardest part right now, and though it seemed tough, it was going to get better.

I assured her that she would get through this trying period and ultimately come to accept the experience as a blessing. I encouraged her to take care of herself—to eat better and exercise—so she could relieve the stress in a healthy way. I hoped she would do a better job of that than I did. I got an email from her yesterday. She told me that she was in a really good place in her life. She was working out regularly and feeling good about how therapy was going with her son. I was encouraged by her words.

If I had the choice, I wouldn't choose for Rhett to have autism. But the Bible says that "in all things God works for the good of those who love him, who have been called according to his purpose" (Romans 8:28). God can even work out a challenging disease like autism for good if you use your experiences to help others.

That's a big reason why I feel my husband and I were chosen to be on *The Biggest Loser*. The moment I got there, I felt strongly in my heart that God had a plan for us that wasn't just about us. Of course, we needed to lose weight so that we could be healthy and set a good example for our families, but I sensed there was more to it than that. I felt God had given my husband and me a greater purpose.

We had always felt as if we were called to be ministers of some sort. We helped out in a church as youth leaders and were also involved in planting a church in Seattle. Although we wanted to be in the ministry, it never seemed to work out as something that we could do full-time. After the final show, I realized that we had been given an opportunity to help others make their lives better, and to top it off, along the way we could share the role our faith played.

Phillip and I didn't win the grand prize, but we won the information we learned to, in turn, teach others. And that is more rewarding than prize money! It has given us the chance to see people live healthier lives and share the source of our strength—our relationship with God.

It Boils Down to Love

Jesus is the ultimate example of a person who thinks about others and puts His own needs aside to fulfill a greater calling. In the book of Luke, we read how Jesus learned about the fate of His close friend, John the Baptist.

John was killed in a gruesome way. Herod was coerced by his mistress, Herodias, to ask her young daughter what she would want for her birthday. Prompted by her mother, the girl requested John the Baptist's head, and so Herod beheaded John, put his head on a platter, and presented it to the daughter as a birthday gift. Herodias hated John because he told Herod that it was not right for him to have a mistress. He had pointed out their sin, and it made Herodias very uncomfortable and ultimately very angry. So Herod did as the girl wished.

"When Jesus heard what had happened [the death of John], he withdrew by boat privately to a solitary place. Hearing of this, the crowds followed him on foot from the towns. When Jesus landed and saw the large crowd, he had compassion on them and healed their sick" (Matthew 14:13-14).

I don't know about you, but if my dear friend was killed, especially in such a horrible way, I would have been full of grief and crumpled up in a fetal position in that "solitary place." I would have probably felt sorry for myself for weeks, cried for just as long, and been consumed by my sorrow. Not Jesus. He went away for a moment, and then, instead of having a pity party, He turned and looked at the needs of the crowd. The Bible tells us He immediately starting healing those who were sick.

In the next part of the story, we find the disciples trying to send the people away because it was getting dark and time for dinner. Despite His aching heart, Jesus told them to let the people stay. Dinner wasn't a problem. He said He could feed them all. I imagine His disciples were confused. They must have looked at Him and thought, *How on earth are we going to prepare dinner for all these people?*

Many of you know what happened next. Jesus took a little boy's lunch of five loaves of bread and two fish and performed the famous miracle of feeding more than five thousand people. He could have easily told the disciples, "Yeah, send the people home, guys. I've had a bad day. I need to rest awhile and be by Myself." After all, He had the perfect out. It was already getting dark, and the people needed to get home to their families anyway.

But He didn't. He let them stay. And He fed them. At a time when He could have chosen to be selfish, Jesus set the example that we all should follow and focused on helping others. You may be thinking, *Come on now. We're talking about Jesus, the Son of God. Of course, it was easy for Him to choose to help others.*

Well, think about this. Jesus was both 100 percent God and 100 percent man. He was tempted with all of the same kinds of things we are tempted with. He loved John, and I am sure He was very sad when he died. I'm sure Jesus had to consciously make the decision to tear away from His time of solitude because of the people's great needs only He could meet. He was motivated because of His love for those He came to die for.

Love is a great motivator. When we love, we sacrifice and put others before ourselves. And we do it with joy, not expecting anything in return but experiencing a fulfillment beyond measure. I'm reminded of a friend who I think is an incredible person. She owns her own business, is a mother of four children, volunteers for various organizations, and through it all maintains a positive and grateful attitude. Just thinking about all she does on a regular basis makes me stressed out!

One day while we were having lunch, she casually told me that she had been a surrogate mother for a friend who couldn't have children. She was so nonchalant about this amazing endeavor, as if she were talking about what she had for dinner the night before. I was touched. What a sacrifice! But my friend didn't see it like that. This precious woman only saw a friend of hers in need and the solution she could offer. It was natural for her to volunteer to carry the child for her friend.

When I think about having a baby, I think about stretch marks, swelling, and the pain of delivery. You make a nine-month commitment to your body. My friend didn't focus on those difficulties. She only thought about blessing her friend.

I cannot tell you how much I admire this friend. Her attitude embodies the practice of love that Jesus has called us to. If she had been too busy thinking about all the responsibilities she had and the challenges she was facing in her own life, she would have never sacrificed her body, time, and so much more—and all that in the name of love.

Being the Difference

The Bible says that all the commandments can be fulfilled by doing two things—love God with all your heart and love your neighbor as yourself (see Matthew 22:37-39). The fit girl understands that this is really what life is all about.

The Bible also tells us there is no greater love than a man who lays down his life for his friend (see John 15:13). I think about all the people in my life who have laid down their lives to help me walk my path in life. While they didn't literally die for me, they gave of themselves in sacrificial ways, so I could live the life God designed for me.

I think about my fifth-grade teacher, Mrs. Gaddy. When I moved to Greer, South Carolina, from Florida, she made me feel like I was her favorite student. She knew I was going through a hard time and that I was a shy kid, so she went out of her way to encourage me and make me feel as if I belonged. She helped me meet friends and made me feel smart even though I was just an average student. I don't know how I would have survived that time in my life if it wasn't for her kind words and support.

I think about the woman who created a scholarship fund that paid my way through Bible college. Her name was Teresa, and she went to my church. When I was in high school, her husband died in a tragic accident. They had three young children. I remember crying my eyes out during his funeral.

Sometime after, Teresa used some of the money she received from his life insurance policy to set up a fund to help people who wanted to go into the ministry. I was one of the recipients. Teresa could have used that money for her own needs (she was now a single mom and had very legitimate needs of her own), but she wanted to sow into the lives of others.

I am so grateful that she gave me the opportunity to learn more about God and His Word. The time I spent at that school changed the course of my life. I will forever be indebted to her act of kindness. Who knows where I would be today if I hadn't received that scholarship? Maybe I wouldn't be sitting here writing this book.

Think about yourself. Have there been people who have sown into your own life? Perhaps they encouraged you at a time you were sinking in depression. Perhaps they gave you financial help when you were down and out. Perhaps they helped you recover from an addiction. Perhaps they even guided you on the path to becoming a fit girl. All these people followed God's call to love Him and others. Doesn't that motivate you to be that kind of person? Doesn't that inspire you to sow into the lives of others?

102 Ways to Focus on Others

1. Help teach a younger child to read.
2. Help cook and/or serve a meal at a homeless shelter.
3. Gather clothing from your neighbors and donate it to a local shelter.
4. Make "I Care" kits with combs, toothbrushes, shampoo, and more for the homeless.

5. Pack and hand out food at a local food bank.

6. Adopt a "grand friend," write them letters, and visit them.

7. Visit senior citizens at a nursing home.

8. Rake leaves, shovel snow, clean gutters, or wash windows for a senior citizen.

9. Pick up groceries or medicine for an elderly person.

10. Go for a walk with a senior citizen in your community.

11. Deliver meals to homebound individuals.

12. Hold an afternoon dance for your local nursing home.

13. Teach a senior friend how to use a computer and the Internet.

14. Paint a mural over graffiti.

15. Invite local police officers to present a drug awareness or safety program.

16. Tutor a student that needs help learning English or another subject.

17. Organize a canned-goods drive.

18. Clean up a vacant lot or park.

19. Organize a campaign to raise money to purchase and install playground equipment.

20. Plant flowers in public areas that could use some color.

21. Volunteer to help at a Special Olympics event.

22. Set up a buddy system for kids with special needs in your community.

23. Raise money for Braille books for visually impaired people.

24. Read books or the newspaper on tape for visually impaired people.

25. Bring toys to children in the cancer ward of a hospital.

26. Contact your local political representative about key issues.

27. Register people to vote.

28. Organize a public issues forum for your neighborhood.

29. Volunteer at a polling booth on election day.

30. Take a friend to the polling booths.

31. Vote.

32. Offer to pass out election materials.

33. Plant a garden or tree where the whole neighborhood can enjoy it.

34. Set up a recycling system for your home.

35. Organize a carpooling campaign in your neighborhood.

36. Adopt an acre of a rainforest.

37. Clean up trash along a river, beach, or in a park.

38. Create a habitat for wildlife.

39. Create a campaign to encourage biking and walking.

40. Test the health of the water in your local lakes, rivers, and streams.

41. Contact your local volunteer center for opportunities to serve.

42. Volunteer at your local animal shelter.

43. Help build a home with Habitat for Humanity.

44. Walk a neighbor's dog or pet sit while they are on vacation.

45. Teach Sunday school.

46. Learn to be a peer counselor.

47. Send a letter to one of America's veterans or overseas soldiers.

48. Volunteer at your local youth center.

49. Participate in a marathon for your favorite charity.

50. Become a volunteer at your local hospital.

51. Mentor a young person.

52. Serve your country by joining AmeriCorps.

53. Become a volunteer firefighter or EMT.

54. Donate books to your local library.

55. Donate clothes to the Salvation Army.

56. Start a book club in your area.

57. Adopt a pet from the Humane Society.

58. Hold a door open for someone.

59. Give up your seat on the bus or train to someone.

60. Donate your old computer to a school.

61. Give blood.

62. Coach a children's sports team.

63. Become an organ donor.

64. Teach a dance class.

65. Participate in Job Shadow Day (February 2).

66. Organize a project for National Youth Service Day.

67. Volunteer to work a hotline.

68. Meet with local representatives from your area.

69. Don't drink and drive.

70. Listen to others.

71. Write a letter to the editor about an issue you care about.

72. Bring others with you when you volunteer.

73. Shop at local, family-owned businesses.

74. Become a Big Brother or Big Sister.

75. Take a historical tour of your community.

76. Write a note to a teacher who had a positive effect on you.

77. Get together with some friends to buy holiday presents for a family at a shelter.

78. Recycle.

79. Drive responsibly.

80. Earn a CPR and First Aid certification.

81. Don't litter.

82. Shop responsibly.

83. Don't spread or start gossip.

84. Tell someone that you appreciate him/her.

85. Hold a teddy bear drive for foster children, fire victims, or other children in need.

86. Make a care package for an elderly or shut-in person.

87. Teach at an adult literacy center.

88. Sing for residents at a nursing home.

89. Befriend a new student or neighbor.

90. Babysit.

91. Look for the good in all people.

92. Coordinate a book drive.

93. Donate money to your favorite charity.

94. Make quilts or baby clothes for low-income families.

95. Bake cookies and take them to your local fire or police station.

96. Donate toys or suitcases to foster children.

97. When visiting someone in a hospital, talk to someone who doesn't have many visitors.

98. During the holidays, visit the post office and answer some letters to Santa.

99. Start a volunteer opportunity in your area.

100. Let the person behind you in the grocery store checkout line go first.

101. Mow the neighbor's lawn for free.

102. Start a neighborhood welcome committee.

When Phillip and I graduated from Bible college, the first ministry opportunity we were offered was to take over a youth group at a small church. We were so excited, and we put our whole hearts into it. We wanted to reach as many kids for God as we could, so we spent our Saturday nights picking up kids in our 1977 blue, two-door Toyota Corolla hatchback from around the neighborhood and taking them to youth group.

We concentrated our efforts on the young people who didn't have parents attending the church and had no way of getting there. Phillip and I wanted to be positive role models to them so they could see God's love through us. It wasn't always easy. Some of these boys and girls were a little rough around the edges.

I remember one such kid; he and his sister had a hard life at home. I could tell that they struggled financially because they were poorly dressed and their house was in bad shape. We weren't sure exactly what their family situation was like, but a lot of conflict seemed to be going on. We made sure to take this particular young man under our wings and love on him in a way that exemplified the love of Christ.

One summer Phillip and I raised money to take the youth group to a Christian youth camp in Florida. We rented vans to haul our ragamuffin group to the southern state for that special week that would change many of their lives. We bonded with these beautiful young people in more ways than we could have ever imagined. The best part was that they all got closer to God. It was a time Phillip and I could sow even more seeds into their lives.

Ten years later, I sat in my office working. I looked up from my desk to see a young man with a scruffy little beard, dirty jeans, and a baseball cap come in. I asked him if I could help him, and he grinned and said, "Don't you recognize me?" To tell you the truth, I didn't.

He laughed and said, "I'm from the youth group." My heart leapt with joy as I jumped up and hugged him. I had finally recognized him as the boy we had taken under our wings so long ago. We talked for a while, catching up on each other's lives. Then he had to go. As he got up to walk out of my office, he said the following words that have since stayed with me, "The year when I came to your youth group was the best year of my life." I almost burst into tears.

You can make a big difference just by loving other people and caring about what is important to them. Phillip and I have kept in contact with several of the kids from that youth group. Today they are a group of good people doing good things with their lives. Some are professionals, worship leaders, youth pastors, devoted wives and husbands, and great fathers and mothers. We feel so blessed to have had a small part in their upbringing.

Mark 8:35 (TLB) says, "Only those who throw away their lives for my sake and for the sake of the Good News will ever know what it means to really live." The Good News is that God sent Jesus as a sacrifice so that we can live eternally. As a fit girl inside and out, you can live the fullest life possible.

Getting fit is not about getting skinny, being admired, or feeling like a beauty queen. Getting fit is not about fitting into your high school jeans or wearing a bikini. Sure, it feels great to be in shape and look the part, but one of the biggest motivators for getting fit should be to impact the lives of others.

Think about particular people or groups you would like to help by donating your time, energy, or resources. How do you want to make a difference in the world? Do you want to start a support group in your community? Sow into the lives of orphans? Work with people with disabilities? Whatever way you want to influence those around you, make that your primary motivation for becoming a fit girl.

My husband's grandfather worked very hard in the beginning of his adult life. He was very successful in the steel business, made wise investments, and was able to retire at an early age. When he retired, he decided to move to Florida and buy a house on the water. All he wanted to do was fish all day.

Eventually he realized there was only so much fishing he could do before he got bored. So he and his wife bought a boat and decided to sail to places they had never been before. They sailed all over the world and brought home wonderful stories of their travels. They even have one about spending Thanksgiving in a cave with a group of fishermen because they had gotten stuck in a storm. They enjoyed traveling for a season, but that got boring too. One day, he was invited to go on a mission trip to Honduras as a lay missionary. He had some construction experience and was able to help build churches in the field.

He loved that trip so much that he took his wife with him the next time. They spent the next several years going back and forth to Honduras. He built churches while she cooked for all the construction workers. It was strenuous, backbreaking work, and it certainly wasn't what you would expect to be doing in your retirement years.

When they were in their nineties, I loved to sit and listen to them talk about their mission work. They said that it was the happiest time in their entire lives. The true joy of their long life came when they knew that they were making a difference in the lives of others.

Philippians 2:3-5 reminds us, "Do nothing out of selfish ambition or vain conceit, but in humility consider others better than yourselves. Each of you should look not only to your own interests, but also to the interests of others. Your attitude should be the same as that of Christ Jesus." What a great truth to live by. Friend, don't make this health journey simply about defeating the fat girl. Make it about the fit girl finding her purpose in making a difference in the lives of others.

TRANSFORMATION TIPS

1. Think about all of the things you could do to help others in a fit body that you can't do in a fat one. Maybe the answer is going on a mission trip that requires a lot of physical labor or having the energy to do more activities with your children. Write these things down.

2. Write a list of the things you find yourself often focusing on. Do you find that those things are the biggest mountains in your life? Maybe you have focused only on your problems or on yourself. If so, think about areas and ways you can shift your attention off of yourself and onto others.

3. Name some people, organizations, or causes you would like to support and help in some way. List the gifts and talents you possess that can be a blessing to them. Make a list of the things you need to adjust in your life so that you can do this. Then go out and do it!

Your Prayer

Father, I pray that You would help me look outside of myself and put my focus on helping other people. Help me follow Your example and put other people's needs ahead of my own. Help me be sensitive to other's hurts and know when I have the ability to help them. In Jesus' name I pray. Amen.

Your Thoughts

Getting Used to the New You

Sow a thought, and you reap an act;
Sow an act, and you reap a habit;
Sow a habit, and you reap a character;
Sow a character, and you reap a destiny.

—Charles Reade

The path to finding the fit girl is a long one wrought with many mental, spiritual, and emotional obstacles, but it's worth it.

Once you find her, the big question is: Now what? I would love to tell you that once you lose the weight and implement all the strategies I talked about in this book, the battle of the fat girl is over. I would love for the new you—the fit girl—to ride into the sunset completely confident and live happily ever after. But fairy tales don't exist. In many ways, once you find the fit girl, a new journey (and sorry, it's not a fairy tale) awaits you. But don't worry; it's ultimately a great adventure. Because I've been through this, I can explain to you what to expect.

When the Fat Girl Doesn't Leave the Building

When I had finished the seven-month process of losing 105 pounds, I took a breath, looked around, and suddenly realized that I didn't know who I was anymore. I had adapted to a role in my life based on my weight. I settled for things that wouldn't have been my first choice. I put myself and my needs last. As a fat girl, I was living a life I wouldn't have necessarily chosen, but I had become quite comfortable in this position.

When I lost the weight, however, things drastically changed. No longer was I the jolly fat friend. I didn't need to overcompensate for my weight by trying to be the life of the party. I didn't take hours to apply my makeup and fix my hair just right so that I wouldn't be embarrassed to go out in public. Dreams I had never imagined were now coming true, and although I appeared as a fit girl doing some wonderful things, I felt uncomfortable in my own skin.

At a time when I should have been jumping for joy over things like shopping for new (nonplus-sized) clothes and having more energy to be physically active, I was feeling out of sorts with this new person. I didn't recognize this fit girl. I didn't know how I should feel, dress, or act because the fat girl did things much differently than the fit girl.

When people asked me, "Amy, don't you feel like a different person?" I could honestly and emphatically say yes. In their minds, feeling like a new person was a good thing, a magical thing, a thing to celebrate. But in my mind, it was quite distressing. I was unsure of what to do with this new person. Being with her was scary and unfamiliar. The fat girl wanted to take a few more breaths before she actually gave up.

It took months for me to adjust my mental image of myself. I took clothes that were much too big into the dressing room, tried them on, and was shocked when they fell right off. I then took a smaller size in, thinking they would never fit, and to my surprise, they fit perfectly. I asked Phillip to point out people who were close to my size because I had no idea how to gauge what I looked like. He got frustrated with me and would say, "Don't you have a mirror?" It didn't matter whether I looked in a mirror or not, I still saw the fat girl looking back at me.

Finally, I started taking pictures of me with friends and family at parties or social events. When I compared my size to those of my skinny friends, I was shocked to find out that I looked just like them size-wise! At first I thought perhaps I was standing in a way that made me look skinnier, or maybe it was an optical illusion. I couldn't believe I was really the size I was.

It took a long time for my mind to catch up to my body. Though I had a fit-girl body, the fat girl was still stuck in my mind.

Seeing the Fit Girl

Making a mental adjustment to the fit-girl mentality is important for two reasons. First, if you hold on to the vision of yourself as the fat girl, you will allow her to be resurrected, and I know that is not what you want.

I have always been a believer that your life follows after your vision. If you see yourself as successful, you'll become more successful. If you believe that you are going to be sick all the time, you'll find yourself in the doctor's office more often. If you continue to see yourself as the fat girl, guess what? You will eventually find that you are the fat girl again.

I did a few things to help transform my vision of myself. I constantly tried on clothes in smaller sizes, I took a lot of pictures of myself, and I weighed and measured myself regularly. I also sought out constant reinforcement from friends and family (particularly from Phillip). Maybe this was a little obsessive and narcissistic, but there was a method to my madness. I wanted to give myself as much evidence as possible to prove that I truly was the fit girl after all. It was the only way I could see myself as her.

Second, it's also important for you to adjust your vision as the new fit girl so you can help someone else who is going through or wants to go through the process. I believe in the "pay it forward" principle. A way to help you heal on your own journey is by helping someone on their journey of healing. If you have been given a gift, you have a responsibility to share it with others. In order to help someone become a fit girl, you first have to believe you are one. If I never saw myself as a fit girl, how could I write a book on becoming one? It would be impossible!

You need to own your new identity and believe that you are never going back to being the fat girl. You have to be adamant that the fat girl is dead and gone! It's the only way you will be able to confidently and powerfully lead others on that same path.

What Do I Wear?

Most women share common challenges when they transform into a fit girl. One of them is not knowing how to dress. This was very true for me. Before I lost weight, I had a certain strategy when it came to buying clothes. My first priority was to find clothes large enough to fit me. Second, I wanted to find colors and prints that were loud in hopes that people would focus more on the clothes than on my fat body.

As a fit girl, those priorities changed. I felt pretty for the first time in a long time, and I wanted to dress the part. The problem was I had a lot of trouble figuring out my style. I didn't know where to begin. There were times (more often than I would like to admit) when I wore clothes that weren't age appropriate. I found myself trying to shop in the junior department even though I was 40 years old. I also wore things that were too short or low cut because now I could wear anything. I wasn't limited to certain styles and sizes, so I took advantage of this newfound freedom.

To be honest, in the beginning of my fashion journey, I probably sent the wrong message with my clothes. I wanted to feel sexy and young, but I ended up looking sleazy and childish. I would have been a perfect candidate for the television show *What Not to Wear*. I can picture the host, Stacey London, shaking her head and saying, "Really?"

Since nothing in my old wardrobe fit, I had to replace everything. I was blessed to have friends and family who gave me clothing they didn't wear anymore. I was especially appreciative because it costs a lot of money to buy new clothes! The only drawback was that my sense of style suddenly looked like it had a multiple-personality disorder. One outfit made me look like my friend; the other made me look like my sister-in-law. You get the idea. I needed to figure out what my new style was apart from looking cheap or like someone else.

I finally had to recruit the help of some friends because I felt that I was incapable of determining this for myself with my skewed self-image. These precious women helped me figure out what looked pretty and modest on me. They helped me get rid of the unflattering clothes and gave me advice on how to compliment my donated wardrobe with new pieces so I could look like me.

Where Do I Fit In?

Trying to figure out my role in social environments was also something that was new for me. For example, before the weight loss process, I had a group of friends I socialized with regularly. I went to parties, movies, and out to dinner with these people.

Occasionally, I went shopping with some of the girls, although I rarely tried on clothes with them because it meant going to separate departments. I was too embarrassed to leave them and go to the plus-sized department, so I would sit with them in the dressing room and give them advice on what looked good or not. We did have common ground as far as shoes and accessories were concerned, and I always tried my best to steer everyone to those particular departments. After all, I've never met a woman who didn't love a pretty pair of shoes! This was one way the fat girl had learned to mask the shame she felt about not being like everyone else.

My husband (who went through a similar transition by becoming a fit guy) and I were always the jolly fat friends and the life of every party. When we went through our weight-loss transformation, we found we were no longer fit (no pun intended) to play those parts. We discovered that our personalities became more subdued. This transition forced us to figure out what our place in our group of friends actually was. The process was especially uncomfortable.

I started receiving a different kind of attention from the opposite sex. As a fat girl, I had always been "one of the guys." As a fit girl, some of my male friends became more flirtatious with me. It was fun being the center of attention for the first time in my life. I would be lying if I said I didn't flirt back a little. But this is not acceptable behavior for a married woman, and I had to come to that truth quickly.

I also had never experienced jealousy from other women. When I became a fit girl, I had a taste of this green-eyed monster from females I once considered my closest friends. Some of them did not even want to associate with me anymore. It hurt. It seemed that as long as I was the fat friend, they liked me. When I lost weight, it was as if these so-called friends felt threatened or just didn't know how I fit into their life anymore.

The process of getting used to the fit girl took time. I had to redis-cover my role—a role that was previously dictated by my weight—with my friends. I was forced to look at who I was and what kind of person I wanted to be. It made me examine so many things about myself that I had never had to think about before.

A lot of good stuff happened through this process. Phillip and I discovered that many of our friends had a social life outside of the en-vironment we knew them in. We knew that our friends socialized on the weekends, but we had no idea that they also socialized during the week at the gym. When we went to the gym for the first time, we were surprised to see our friends there. They had never talked about work-ing out around us because they assumed that since we were overweight, we wouldn't be interested in fitness.

This discovery added a new layer to our relationships—a good layer! Suddenly, rather than just having dinner or going to parties, we could now play racquetball or go to spin classes with them. Many of our friends were avid runners, and we all signed up for a couple of races together. This part of the journey of accepting the fit girl was a beautiful and encouraging thing to me. It definitely made me feel more at ease in my new role!

Warning: Keep Things in Perspective

I believe that many fat girls don't transition fully into fit girls be-cause it feels safer, securer, and more comfortable to stay as they are. I can understand why recovering alcoholics fall off the wagon and peo-ple in abusive relationships stay with their abuser. It's easier to return to what you know than to venture into a world that is relatively unknown.

Many are so afraid to explore this uncharted territory that they wonder, *How do I know things will be better? They may be worse for all I know! Even though I am living a life that is not what I want, at least I know what to expect.* Can you relate?

Life without surprises or changes is familiar, predictable, and com-fortable. When you lose weight, life changes in many ways. Much of the familiar is gone. It's like opening up Pandora's box. It makes you think about every area of your life. You come face-to-face with the realization that you have missed out on so many things as a result of being overweight. You uncover this new person, and the world seems wide open with new possibilities.

It's an amazing feeling, but it can also be dangerous. When you transform into a fit girl, you have to keep a realistic perspective. I know many who have lost a lot of weight and began questioning where they were in their marriage, career, and life. Many people feel as though they'd settled for less; that they'd been so comfortable for such a long time. Now they have access to this brand new world, and they want to get rid of their old life. In some ways, this can be healthy (like getting rid of unhealthy hobbies, negative thoughts, or bad habits).

In other ways, however, it can be a bad thing. Let me explain. Becoming a fit girl can cause tension in your family because they now have to look at you and relate to you in a new way. These adjustments can produce discontent—especially in a marriage. Some people find the conflict so great that they are tempted to abandon relationships rather than stick with them and grow through the process.

I know a lady who recently lost a great deal of weight. She is (and always was) beautiful and has a renewed sense of self-confidence. She shared with me that she had been struggling in her marriage since she had lost weight. The problem, she explained, is that she had always done everything for her children and husband. She felt like a self-made martyr because she made a habit out of putting herself last. Their wish was her command at the expense of her identity.

Once she lost the weight, she felt as though she was getting this great new lease on life. She wanted her family to share in her success and be excited for her. Unfortunately, she received the opposite reaction. She actually felt like her husband wished she was heavy again. Her losing weight brought out all of his insecurities.

When she was heavy, he didn't worry about her doing anything else besides taking care of him and the kids. When she became a fit girl, however, she became empowered. She understood that she needed some time for herself every day to work out and take care of herself emotionally, mentally, physically, and spiritually. This made her husband feel as if she was slipping away from him.

Her transformation also required him to help more with the kids so that she could have that time to tend to her needs. She now needed her children to take on more responsibility as well. As you can imagine, her husband and kids rebelled against all these changes. They liked it when Mom took care of everything for them. I mean, wouldn't you? My friend had to work through this transition instead of doing what is tempting to most people—throw in the towel and start a new life.

Another friend of mine told me that after she lost weight, her husband became extremely jealous. The funny thing was that there was no reason for it. She didn't solicit the attention of other men or even react when they gave it to her. Her husband simply started to notice that she was getting more looks than she had been given before, and it made him extremely insecure. He began to monitor her phone calls and text messages. He constantly questioned her whereabouts—even when she went to the grocery store. He called her throughout the day to check up on her.

For the first time in her marriage, my friend felt as if she was under surveillance 24 hours a day. Instead of being a husband, her spouse became a private investigator. No matter what she did, she couldn't convince him that she had no interest in other men and that she only wanted to be with him. His insecurity convinced him that she was going to leave him any minute. I can only imagine that this environment would make anyone want to run back to the safety of the fat girl.

Here's another challenge you might face as a fit girl. You might find yourself questioning if where you live or what you do for a living is what you really want now. You may find that where you live is not a community that supports your new active lifestyle. For instance, you might want to move somewhere with more access to parks, walking trails, or recreational activities.

You might even find that your job is too sedentary for you. As a fat girl, you may have taken a job that didn't involve much activity because your weight was an issue. As a fat girl, you might not have had the confidence to apply for the job you really wanted because your weight held you back. Perhaps you were judged for being overweight. Many employers associate extra pounds with laziness. While this is a false assumption, sadly it is a mind-set that many people espouse. You may feel lost in your career and in a position you have to rethink or even reinvent.

Changes don't stop at marriage and career. If you have children, what about them? Perhaps you struggle with guilt because you have wasted a lot of time as a fat girl and even missed out on precious moments with your kids because of the extra weight. All these things are part of the potential growing pains involved with getting used to the new you. Be encouraged. It is possible to work through all these issues and embrace and enjoy the new you. Read books, see a therapist, and talk to other people who have similar struggles. Do what you have to do to start looking at yourself, appreciating what you see, and living your life as a fit girl.

Sometimes it's hard to move forward as a fit girl because you are tied down by regrets. I know a lot about them. When my children were little and I was a fat girl, I rode an emotional roller coaster. I believe it was because my blood sugar was a mess due to the way I ate. I used to wake up in the morning, drink coffee, and run out the door. I went for hours without eating because I wanted to save my calories for later in the day. By the time I did eat, I was so famished that I didn't care about calories anymore. I just wanted food—and lots of it! The food gave me temporary energy, but an hour later, I crashed.

The crash usually coincided with the time my kids came home from school. I used to dread this time of day because I needed to have energy to make snacks for them, pack lunches for the next day, change them out of their school clothes and into their play clothes, and do homework with them. I was so tired; however, that all I wanted to do was to take a nap.

With three small children running around, a nap was out of the question. So I tried to give myself a boost with more coffee or energy drinks just to get through the afternoon. All it did was make me grumpy. I was always in a bad mood during this time and yelled at my kids nonstop. My poor little boys!

I look back with some regret. I wish I had known then what I know now! But isn't that the case with life? As a fit girl, I can't waste my time and well-being thinking about how I could have done things better. All I can do is focus on the things I can do now with my children. The awesome part of being a fit girl is that I have energy to do things with them that I never did before. We can go to an amusement park, and I can walk around all day. When we go on vacation, I don't have to just stay in the hotel room; I can run on the beach. These are positive aspects of the transformation I made sure to focus my attention on.

What About Plastic Surgery?

Another part of getting used to the new you has to do with something I am often asked about. If I had a dollar for every time a woman came up to me after hearing me speak and sheepishly asked me the following questions, I would have quite a nest egg. The questions are: What do you do about the loose skin? Did you have to have surgery? Everyone is curious about that, and those are valid questions that deserve answers.

When you lose a large amount of weight, you end up with skin that has been stretched out and now sags. If you are in your twenties or thirties and have never had children, there is a chance your skin has enough elasticity to bounce back, and you won't have the skin problem. If you are 40 or older and have had children, then you may not be able to get rid of the loose skin without plastic surgery.

I lost my weight when I was 40 and as of now have not had any plastic surgery. I have consulted with a plastic surgeon, and he told me that because I did a lot of weight training, I had much less skin on my arms and legs than someone who might not have weight trained. He told me that some of my areas of concern, which are my abdomen and breasts, would never bounce back because I have had three children and am over 40. He also said that the muscle tone under the loose skin was good, and so if I elected to have a procedure, I would have an easier time because he wouldn't have to cut into my muscles to tighten them up.

I have not decided whether or not I will do it. I wrestle back and forth between whether or not I should. One part of me says that I should do it to get rid of the remnants of the fat girl once and for all. I know that I would be able to run better without it around my waist. The other part of me questions whether the money I would have to spend could be better used for a nobler and less vain purpose. Don't get me wrong. I am not opposed to plastic surgery. I feel that if a woman wants to do that, it is her choice. She knows her financial situation and her motives.

In some cases having that sagging skin is a real problem. Because of the constant rubbing, rashes and sores can develop and have a hard time healing. Excess skin between the legs and under the arms can impair movement. In these situations, I would encourage you to consult with a surgeon, knowing that insurance companies often pay for the surgery under these circumstances. If you feel that surgery will boost your self-confidence and help you realize your full potential, then I encourage you to talk to a surgeon about your options. People don't always choose plastic surgery for vain reasons. Sometimes they truly need it.

Change Is Good

Changing from a fat girl to a fit girl takes time. Some parts of the process may not be pleasant, but it's necessary and worth it. It took seven months for me to lose the weight and seven more months to deal with the emotional issues that followed. I believe the last seven months were just as important—if not more important—than the first seven months.

You may have lost weight and gained it back a hundred times. Maybe the journey after losing the weight was what tripped you up. It's very possible because this second part is what nobody really talks about. It's not fun, and it's a lot of work. But it's also the final scene in setting the stage for your new act as a fit girl. This is where you move toward owning your new identity. When you lose the weight, you will find yourself at a crossroads (you might even be there already) where you have to make the final decision—am I going to run forward to the fit-girl life or turn around and run back to the fat-girl life.

I can tell you from experience that the longer I embraced the fact that I was no longer the fat girl, the fit girl got stronger. Soon enough I stopped being afraid that the fat girl was going to come back. I was finally able to realize I had the power to ensure that she was gone forever.

I hear stories all the time from people who have lost a great deal of weight, but before they know it, those lost pounds creep back up. When I talk to them, I usually find that pressure and stress have entered their life, and rather than face it, they run back to the habits that brought them comfort. These comforts are what sabotaged them to begin with and gave the fat girl control.

I want to encourage you! You have the power to prevent that from happening. You have the ability to embrace the new you rather than let the fat girl regain control. Realize the benefits of being a fit girl and start getting excited for your new fit future.

There are dreams inside of you that are dying to be resurrected. There are things you once thought impossible that can now be a reality. The limitations you used to set on yourself are gone. As a fit girl, you are free to live the life God has planned for you—a life that is full of blessing, fulfillment, peace, and meaning. That life is abundant and designed uniquely for you. Get used to this new life and turn away from the old one. It's time to enjoy your life, fit girl!

⊱ TRANSFORMATION TIPS ⊰

1. Think about the challenges you may encounter when you reach your goal weight. If you have already lost a lot of weight, list some of the challenges you are currently facing.

2. In what areas of your life have you settled for less? Maybe you have a special talent you've kept dormant and hidden out of fear of having to use it. Do you have dreams locked up in your heart that have never been realized because of your weight? Maybe you wanted to travel through Europe or start a new career. Write them down.

3. How do you think your weight loss will affect these areas of your life—relationships, career, home, and so forth?

4. List some steps you can take to prevent going back to your old life. For example, you could talk with a therapist or try to meet and support others who are in a similar situation as you are.

⊱ Your Prayer ⊰

Father, help me live my life as a fit girl. Keep me from running back to the comforts of the fat girl. I know this transformation is not easy and that when I lose weight, some changes might be uncomfortable. Help me stay grounded in my new life and mind-set so that I may glorify You. I pray that You would reveal to me the exciting new life I can live as a fit girl. Teach me to embrace this part of the journey. In Jesus' name I pray. Amen.

Your Thoughts

Stay connected with Amy online at
www.philandamyfitness.com

Get the latest updates on her speaking schedule,
media appearances, and more by visiting her

Twitter address: @philandamy
Facebook fan page: Phil and Amy Fitness

To inquire about Amy speaking at your
women's group or church, please contact

JChaffee@chaffeemanagement.com

To learn more about other Harvest House books
or to read sample chapters, log on to our website:
www.harvesthousepublishers.com

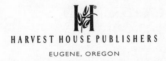

HARVEST HOUSE PUBLISHERS
EUGENE, OREGON

Begin Your Own Journey to Becoming a Fit Girl

THE 90-DAY FITNESS CHALLENGE
by Phil and Amy Parham

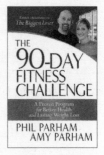

Phil and Amy Parham, contestants on NBC's *The Biggest Loser,* provide a faith-based, informative, and motivational book that will encourage you to face your weight challenges, permanently transform your life, and live your dream of being healthier, happier, and more fit.

This is not a diet book for temporary change but a manual for permanent transformation. *The 90-Day Fitness Challenge* will

- encourage you to embark on a 90-day program for permanent weight loss
- outline simple and practical healthy food and fitness plans
- point the way toward developing better eating habits and an active lifestyle
- incorporate Scripture and faith principles to encourage you to make God a part of your journey
- provide motivation through heartfelt and encouraging daily devotional readings

The Parhams know from personal experience the obstacles to fitness that you face. Having lost a combined total of 256 pounds, they come alongside you to provide inspiration, motivation, and practical life skills on their 90-day journey toward better health and lasting weight loss.

THE 90-DAY FITNESS CHALLENGE DVD
by Phil and Amy Parham

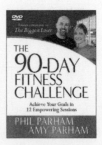

The Parhams bring their inspiring, you-can-do-it style on-screen, presenting the Challenge in twelve 15-minute sessions (180 minutes total). Along with cooking and exercise tips, they emphasize practical food plans, changes in eating habits, and development of an active lifestyle, all based on biblical principles. *Two DVDs; for individuals or groups.*